Issues and Concepts in Patient Education

Issues and Concepts in Patient Education

Barbara Klug Redman, Ph.D., Editor
Professor (On Leave), School of Nursing
University of Colorado Health Sciences Center
Denver, Colorado

Contributors

Nancy Lloyd Rothman, R.N., M.Ed., M.S.N.
Assistant Professor, Villanova University
Villanova, Pennsylvania

Daniel A. Rothman, J.D.
Adjunct Faculty, Gwynedd Mercy College
Gwynedd Valley, Pennsylvania

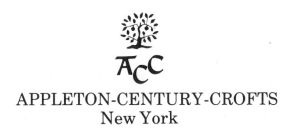

APPLETON-CENTURY-CROFTS
New York

81 82 83 84 85 / 10 9 8 7 6 5 4 3 2 1

Prentice-Hall International, Inc., London
Prentice-Hall of Australia, Pty. Ltd., Sydney
Prentice-Hall of India Private Limited, New Delhi
Prentice-Hall of Japan, Inc., Tokyo
Prentice-Hall of Southeast Asia (Pte.) Ltd., Singapore
Whitehall Books Ltd., Wellington, New Zealand

Library of Congress Cataloging in Publication Data

Redman, Barbara Klug.
  Issues and concepts in patient education.

  (Patient education series)
  Bibliography: p.
  Includes index.
  1. Patient education.   2. Nurse and patient.
I. Title. II. Series.
RT90.R4   610.73   80-25782
ISBN 0-8385-4405-3

Text design: Karin Batten
Cover design: Gloria Moyer
Cover photography: Robert Goldstein

PRINTED IN THE UNITED STATES OF AMERICA

Introduction to the Patient Education Series

A great deal of development has occurred in patient education in the last decade. Programs are much more widespread; valuable experience has been gained in applying general educational theory and practice in many areas of clinical practice.

It seemed propitious to reflect that development in a series of books aimed at sharing the emerging body of knowledge gained by practitioners in specialized fields. The authors are pioneers in developing practical tools to evaluate and document patient learning. The emphasis is on clinical usability, focusing on patient assessment for desired behavior, educational interventions, evaluation and outcome criteria, and recording. Also in the series is a book on issues and concepts in patient education with an abbreviated review of teaching, learning and motivation theory, and a focus on issues I perceive to be important in the development of the field. A second book focuses on examples of strategies for institutional change and of systems for delivery of patient education. Strategies of this kind have been very important in dealing with systems that have been resistant and unresponsive to incorporation of patient education into practice.

Producing the series has been educative for those involved. By history and tradition, patient education has been better developed conceptually and more completely accepted and incorporated into some clinical areas than into others. One realizes that this has sometimes occurred because of patterns of delivery of services and because of the predominant medical approaches to problems, and not necessarily on the basis of patient need and ability to profit from education. I hope that the series helps to identify areas needing development and that the imaginative clinicians with whom we are blessed will find the ideas of use in further maturation of the field.

It is important not to underestimate the significance of the patient education movement. Along with other related practices and philosophies, it reflects a very basic change in the standard of care and in the relationship between providers and clients. Like all basic changes, its processes for development are sometimes agonizingly slow and are conglomerations of rational and political processes, and its structures are often loosely coupled and disconnected. However, the movement does reflect the commitment of many lay people and professionals who believe patient education yields more humane care and is also effective as a treatment modality.

A word must be said about the contribution to the series of Leslie Boyer at Appleton-Century-Crofts. The series was her idea, and she was a major partner in its development at every stage.

BARBARA KLUG REDMAN
Washington, D.C.

Each individual should have the opportunity to learn about preventive and corrective health problems. Therefore, every health profession and nursing in particular must incorporate health teaching into its practice whether the client is an individual, a family or a community.

Barbara Redman's discussion of health education is timely and lucid. She not only gives nurses the information they need to deliver health care, but also provides them with the means to evaluate its effectiveness.

The American Nurses' Association believes professional nurses are responsible and accountable for quality nursing care. This includes teaching patients about specific health care needs and supporting appropriate modifications of behavior. The books in this series should be useful tools to help them fulfill their increasing responsibilities in this area.

Barbara Nichols, President
American Nurses' Association

Foreword

It is a special honor to share a few thoughts with you on the first of the 13 books in this landmark series on the subject of in-hospital and ambulatory patient education.

Patient teaching in various forms has been on the scene for the greater part of this century. But it was the demonstration projects and studies which began in the 1940s and the invitational conferences sponsored by the American Hospital Association that provided the theoretical framework on which many of today's patient education programs are modeled. The Presidential Commission on Health Education in 1972 helped pave the way for the present unparalleled interest in disease prevention and health promotion on the part of the general public, business, industry, government, health care providers, and schools. A commission task force prepared a paper on *The Concept of Planned, Hospital-Based Patient Education Programs* that has been widely circulated. Other important developments were the release of a statement by the American Nurses' Association on *The Professional Nurse and Health Education,* the expansion of the American Hospital Association's focus on patient education to a broader health promotion thrust, and, under contract with the Bureau of Health Education, an analysis of a nationwide hospital survey on in-patient education.

Recent federal legislation has either alluded to or called for health education services: the Health Maintenance Organization Assistance Act of 1973 (PL93-22) and the National Health Planning and Resources Development Act of 1974 (PL93-641). And, in a similar vein, the Joint Commission on the Accreditation of Hospitals will soon require institutions to meet its standards for patient education programs.

Soaring health care expenditures, $202.3 billion in 1979—a 13 percent increase over 1978 and a staggering 8.5 percent proportion of the gross national product—affect everyone. These rising costs have, in fact, sparked a national cost containment movement, with the concept of health promotion an important part of that movement.

Cost-effective patient education services that are integral to quality patient care will be looked to. And to furnish these services various partnerships will increasingly be necessary, on the part of providers, consumers, business, industry, community health resources, and third party payers.

Formalized referral linkages must emerge and barriers to programs must be countered. New and different disciplines, such as health economics, will be called upon by both providers and insurers. New sites for health promotion and patient education programs will evolve. I'm thinking, for example, of the emerging programs at the worksite and increased national interest in school health education. And, of course, more continuing education will be needed to provide health professionals with the appropriate skills and knowledge about the latest educational methodologies, communication techniques, and technology.

We are clearly in the midst of a social change of major proportions. As we approach the year 2000, we must build on the excellent studies, demonstration projects and resources that are already in place. We have an increasingly well-informed citizenry of all ages, who will expect, and should receive, quality preventive, secondary, and tertiary health care services.

One of the basic assumptions of the Trends Analysis Program of the American Council on Life Insurance was: "The Future is not beyond our control, what we do today will affect the future; we are not at the mercy of totally unpredictable or pre-ordained decisions." While some will debate the latter, and rightfully so, I can think of no better example of the underlying validity of this assumption than the dramatic decline in mortality from cardiovascular disease in the United States—down some 22 percent in the last decade (1968-77). This decrease has been attributed, in part, to extensive health education efforts concerning known risk factors such as hypertension, smoking, and high cholesterol levels, as well as to improved detection, diagnostic techniques, and medical care.

Patient education is clearly an idea whose time has come. It is a process that needs to be elevated to a position of major consideration by all, with a role in health care. Not only can it hasten recovery and reduce the number of hospitalizations and re-admissions, it is, above all, the humane way to proceed.

L. Virginia Fernbach, M.A.
Health Education Administrator
Health and Safety Education Division
Metropolitan Life Insurance Company
Chairwoman, Task Force on Patient Education
Presidential Commission on Health Education

Preface

This book started as an attempt to simplify the confusing content about teaching and learning in patient education. Like all supposedly simple tasks, it was in reality very complex.

How much of the learning literature is useful in a practical health situation, especially for patient education as opposed to school education? Writing this book has helped to clarify for the author how different patient education is from school education and how inappropriate is the not uncommon mixing of the models in patient education practice. The goals are different: cognitive skill and discipline-oriented for the school model versus independent handling of a health behavior for patient education, which often requires neither knowledge of a discipline nor high-level cognitive skills. The methods likely to be useful are also then different and require for patient education the development of methods that are good for teaching problem solving in an irregular time frame. Management of the environment to support learning is expected in the school but not in patient education, even though instructionally potent events are occurring frequently. Among health professionals is a general lack of conscious awareness that patient education can create negative side effects, although that concept is well understood in schools. The goal in patient education is usually not seen as distant as in school education but is more immediate and practical, such as compliance with a regimen. Toward such an all-important goal, many kinds of strategies to change behavior are used, teaching often being intermixed with other strategies.

Also deeply affecting its practice is the fact that patient education is part of the health care system and represents only one of the goals of that system. It is unlikely that its goals will suddenly become predominant, that superb learning conditions will be created, or that learning will be seen as a useful goal in itself.

The book is meant to be supportive of the other books in the series through discussion of issues and concepts basic to the whole field. The focus is not primarily on the process of teaching, which is explained in the health condition specialty books in the series. This introductory book does, however, interpret the field and make prescriptions for it in ways that may well not be agreeable to all participating in this endeavor.

I hope that this book will be useful for practice and that this is accomplished through a clearer conceptualization than has been available in the past of the differences from school learning, and the interrelationships with other strategies in the health care setting.

BARBARA KLUG REDMAN
Potomac, Maryland

Table of Contents

1

PATIENT EDUCATION: TEN ERRONEOUS ASSUMPTIONS

Erroneous assumptions about some basic relationships between patient teaching and patient learning are common. Sometimes this state of affairs represents a misconception or a misunderstanding. In other instances, the true relationship is understood in discussion, but in practice the erroneous assumption is carried out. In general, the force of these erroneous assumptions is to weaken teaching and, at the same time, to create unrealistic expectations about its outcomes.

Characteristically, the most commonly suggested way to correct the erroneous assumptions is to teach patient educators "the facts." This is one approach, but it ignores the need for patient educators to gain skill in putting good practice into operation, which often requires a change in what "the system" allows and rewards.

1. A patient learns what he has been told. Everyone, based on common sense, knows that people often do not retain or even understand what they have been told. The stress of health situations often results in even less comprehension. Yet, telling continues in many health situations and therefore misassumptions are frequently put into operation. Misunderstanding probably occurs for several reasons. It is assumed that the patient will make an extraordinary effort to comprehend the health information that the provider feels is important. It takes time and patience to obtain repeated feedback from the patient to make sure he understands what may be a very complicated topic. And there are real problems with translating medical jargon to lay people. Finally, the provider may believe that a dominant authoritarian relationship with his client is appropriate and that part of this relationship involves the patient accepting whatever the provider says. Educating a patient requires much more effort and skill in working past learning problems than just having the patient comply with a series of commands.

Standards of care seem to be rapidly moving toward requirement of patient understanding and ability to perform when the patient is able and willing. For this reason, patient education operations in which telling is the dominant mode, without adequate feedback to determine level of understanding, will not be acceptable.

2. Patient learning in health environments occurs exclusively or primarily when he is being "taught," usually in a formal setting like a class.   Just being in a health care environment is often a very potent educational experience for patients. Imagine the patient seeing another patient in the next bed resuscitated from a cardiac arrest. Parents of children with diabetes or leukemia often learn from each other in a waiting room. There are numerous such examples to which patients are often very sensitive because they are vulnerable in a health crisis. Such experiences can be erroneous and not well integrated in the patient's mind while chance experiences usually do not constitute a complete educational experience. Obviously, a professional teaching responsibility is to help patients make such experiences constructive.

Interactions and settings perceived by the patient as informal often create the most learning. Formal student–teacher settings in classrooms using such devices as tests often frighten patients. For this reason, teaching them as part of the normal interaction while care is being given is often very effective. Planned use of the environment, e.g., putting a patient with another from whom he will learn, or assisting a naturally formed social group of mothers in the waiting room, is also effective. No one really knows how much patient teaching and learning goes on informally, nor do we really know the extent to which it is positive or negative. But for a number of reasons (see Chap. 2), the formal school model is not optimal for patient education.

3. Knowledge about a disease significantly affects the patient's compliance with the treatment regimen for that disease.   The scientific evidence on the relationship between compliance and knowledge is clearly not all in. What is clear is that compliance and noncompliance are highly complex behaviors affected by a wide range of factors. Such factors include complexity of the regimen, relationship with the health care provider including degree of supervision, family stability, and health beliefs of the individual. At present, at least one summary of the research indicates little or no relationship between patient knowledge of the disease and its therapy and the compliance with the associated treatment regimen.[1] While compliance with a regimen is a goal commonly desired by health care providers, its definition as an instructional goal is far from clear. Absolute blind adherence to a regimen can be dangerous. Certainly, at least in selected patients, intelligent compliance with ability to stop or adjust the regimen is more useful. Even in situations where the regimen is usually effective, the degree of compliance required is not always clear. Can one get protection from recurrence of rheumatic fever by taking only a portion of the prescribed prophylactic penicillin?[1]

The chance of affecting compliance seems to be greater with use of a wide range of behavior change strategies besides the usual counseling and fact-teaching approaches. Simplification of medication schedules, increased supervision of the patient, convenient clinics, and so forth are useful.[1]

4. Knowing "why" is necessary for knowing "how." In many ways, it is useful to think of "why" information as a separate but related body of knowledge from that related to "how." It is common to think that both bodies of knowledge are necessary to teach to a patient, and at times a greater emphasis is placed on "why." Indeed, some degree of "why" knowledge is important for informed consent, and in some people it serves as a motivator, giving them a feeling of control over a frightening illness. But an overemphasis on "why" can replace skill training: a patient may know about his disease but not be skilled in carrying out his regimen or integrating it into his life. Often teaching "why" to an intelligent patient is easier than hammering out with him how he will alter his life and habits to live with a chronic disease.

Another danger of "why" oriented instructional programs is that they can be used as artificial means of screening people out of instructional programs that are critical to their well-being. It is not always necessary to understand the scientific principles on which equipment or treatment is based in order to treat oneself successfully.

5. Educational interventions do not include assisting the patient to learn how to carry out the desired behavior in life or an alteration of the environment such as change in clinic schedules to shorten waiting time. The environment actually gives very strong educational messages. Patient teaching often is associated with a very narrow range of intervention strategies, primarily those aimed at giving the patient factual knowledge. Other strategies may be called behavioral or psychosocial. The broad field of education has always combined all of these strategies, including manipulation of the environment, to support performance of the desired behavior. In school, perhaps the educational emphasis has been on cognitive learning since that has been a strong priority of schools as institutions. A related area of confusion in the health field has been the differences and similarities between the theories and therapies of psychiatry and those of teaching and other psychosocial interventions. This topic is addressed in Chapter 7.

6. Until a patient indicates he is ready, he will not learn. Everyone knows that a person has to be willing to learn. This is embodied in the old saying, "You can lead a horse to water, but you can't make him drink." Readiness to learn, especially about one's health, is an area that is not well documented with scientific evidence. Perhaps the problem arises when the health care provider decides to wait for the patient to initiate a request for teaching. Readiness is assumed to be the responsibility of the patient, and he is to communicate it as openly and as directly as possible. By taking this attitude, the professional abdicates the responsibility for influencing readiness. Natural readiness to learn does occur, and its presence should be monitored and recognized by the provider. For example, because of a crisis in their lives (deterioration of a parent with emphysema), persons (the parent's teenage children) sometimes feel vulnerable and may be ready to change behavior (smoking cessation). Psychosocial adaptation to an illness occurs in phases, each with a natural readiness, so a patient who is in rehabilitation after a myocardial infarction may be more ready to consider the necessary life changes than he was when in a stage of denial right after diagnosis.

Readiness can also be stimulated in a patient by several strategies related to giving him a perception of control over what is happening to him. One such strategy is to teach him what he wants to know first. Another is to teach him in an unobtrusive way the techniques and skills he needs to control his situation. In patients who respond more readily to authoritative demands rather than to internal desires to know, readiness can be stimulated by the authority issuing a demand.

7. Attitudes have to be changed before behavior will change. Usually, the goal of health education is a change of behavior in a patient, such as performing regular breast self-examination. If a patient did not feel positively about doing breast self-examination, it was assumed that the proper strategy was to persuade her to change her attitudes and that the desired behavior would then follow. The relationship between attitude and behavior is complex and certainly not well understood. But often attitude change occurs if the patient is first assisted to do the desired behavior.

8. A written plan for teaching intervention bears some resemblance to what occurs. A written plan that often is carried out by many persons must have at least two characteristics to be reliably implemented: terms with commonly understood meanings and accountability for the activity. Patient education often has neither.

With an adequate level of teaching skill, one nurse providing continuity of care can probably more effectively teach a patient than will many nurses who work briefly with him. Since there are many teaching strategies, it is easier for the nurse to follow his or her own plan than to try to carry out someone else's. For some patients, differences in language, affect, and other instructional strategies are confusing. The inability of the recently assigned nurse to pick up behavioral cues that the former nurse was able to detect can mean opportunity missed or behavior misinterpreted. If health professionals are not accountable for assessment of the adequacy of patient behavior and for assisting with change when necessary, instructional opportunities are often not made available, and other activities simply take priority.

9. Once a patient has learned "the basics" about a health condition or a behavior he is to perform, he generally requires little additional education, and what he does require he can generally obtain for himself informally. Educational programs are predominantly aimed at assisting people with initial learning. Perhaps this is so because the need for education at that time is obvious and can be fairly standardized since most people start with little knowledge. Less well-documented is the need for reteaching, sometimes to combat forgetting and decline of motivation, but also to provide new skills in dealing with problems, life stresses, and changes in self-concept which arise as one manages a chronic illness over time. Initial learning programs can be useful for review and update but may well be unsatisfactory in addressing all needs.

10. Physical care always has a higher priority than does patient education. This is, again, an operational error in some settings rather than a misconception. Many nurses can indicate times when a patient's need for information and skills was acute causing anguish or physical danger. For less immediate patient education needs, such as preventive education in which the risk of the occurrence of the problem to be prevented is moderate, priorities with physical care often are not even addressed. Commonly, physical care and teaching are seen as two nonrelated categories of care. Even if both categories of care are being performed, there usually is not clear thinking about and comparison of the relative benefits of various elements of physical care and of the progress toward meeting behavioral goals that might be made through teaching.

REFERENCES

1. Sackett, D. L., & Haynes, R. B. (Eds.). *Compliance with therapeutic regimens.* Baltimore: The Johns Hopkins University Press, 1976.

2

THE SCHOOL MODEL: ITS LIMITATIONS FOR PATIENT EDUCATION

The health care system plays a significant role as educator of its clients, even though that potential has had limited recognition and value. Most major institutions in society have an educative, socializing, or acculturating function about which they are more or less conscious. As the institution formally assigned a primarily educational role, the school has developed a model of educating that is more or less applicable to other institutions.

This chapter addresses two points. First, it characterizes the present patient education model, the way in which the health care system views its educative responsibilities and carries them out. Second, it compares that model with the school model and elucidates the errors made when that school model is used in patient education. The vagueness surrounding the patient education effort often means that a distinctive model is not seen for that effort; the health care worker simply applies the model he knows best, from the school.

CHARACTERIZATION OF PRESENT PATIENT EDUCATION PRACTICE

One is struck by how subordinate the educative task has been to the dominant goal of treatment and the ethos that the physician should control when and if the patient will learn. If there has been a major behavior pattern for the patient in the health care system, it has been compliance, i.e., whether the patient followed the physician's orders. The greatest legal base of concern has been that of informed consent. The flow of influence has been seen as one way from the care giver to the patient with little consideration of how the patient influences and educates the care-giver and affects the system.

The nature of educative tasks in health ranges from a crucial, complex life-saving skill (e.g., home hemodialysis), basic change in life pattern (e.g., altering coronary risk behaviors), to simple information retention. Patients vary in their ability to learn, based on physiological and psychological health, and basic intellectual capacity and learning skills.

Unlike the family acting as educator, the health care system consists of a series of transient environments, often only vaguely coherent in their educative messages. A large proportion of patient education is done on an informal one-to-one basis by health care professionals usually under severe time constraints, with neither in-depth coverage of the instructional material nor follow-up.[3] Patients from a low socioeconomic class may experience difficulty in learning because of a distinct difference in style from that of health care professionals. In most health care environments, very few educative methodologies are available, and in the absence of tried and effective tools almost unreasonable burdens are placed on the interpersonal skills and the time of care-givers.

There is considerable conceptual separation among quite distinct realms of health education. What is taking place in schools is different from public health education, and different also from patient education as part of curative health services. There is a limited body of theory, such as the Health Belief Model, which explains predisposition to take health action, and is apparently useful for a wide variety of health learning.[1]

THE SCHOOL AND PATIENT EDUCATION MODELS

The author's conception of these two models is shown in Table 2-1. From the comparison, both some differences and some deficiencies in the patient education model become clear.

Following are some errors that can occur in patient education emanating from these deficiencies or from inappropriate use of the school model for patient education.

1. Confusion in content and goals between learning a discipline and using a variety of content to alter a living behavior.   The classic example of this confusion is the physician teaching differential diagnosis of asthma to a group of parents of asthmatic children, whose real task is not to learn how to do a differential diagnosis. It is not unusual for a health professional to fall back into teaching the content, often in the way in which he was taught. This occurs particularly if the health professional has not thought through the skills the patient must have and those he does not need.

2. Ambivalence about basic learning skills and maturation.   The health care system rarely has in its consciousness its collective and accumulative impact on a patient other than for his medical condition. Its deliberate educational interventions are short-term (at least the intervention is short-term if not the intended behavior change). Rarely is the intervention deliberately focused on producing maturation, so it does not look for such effect it may have had, either positive or negative. It is probably impossible to move through a health crisis without maturational impact, and the chances for positive development in that situation may not be utilized.

The confusion and narrow vision regarding the long-term learning effects of

TABLE 2-1.
COMPARISON OF SCHOOL AND PATIENT EDUCATION MODELS

Model Elements	School Model	Patient Education Model
Task	Learn cultural knowledge to the skill of problem solving.	Alter a basic living behavior. There is avoidance of basic learning or thinking-skill development.
Curricular focus	A discipline such as history, or a group of basic skills such as reading.	Information and skills are selected and organized around the health behavior to be changed. Usually, a combination of medical knowledge and living skills is used as a conceptual framework.
Political base	Recognized.	Not recognized. Teaching activity may be receiving more attention because of political need to "share" power with the public than because of real conviction of its therapeutic effectiveness. The value base of medicine has not been seriously threatened. Education as a discipline has not been a potent force—witness the considerable lag of application of practice known by that discipline to be effective and the disconnection from school health education.
Learner's motivational base	There is a societal mandate to go to school. The school itself uses certain reinforcers.	There is a variety of motivational bases, but all may be missing in any one patient: A. Personal style and standard of coping B. Health authority mandate (usually physician), although law mandates some behaviors C. Behavior change may be reinforced by lessening of symptoms
	The institution can interfere with a desirable motivational base.	Same as school model.
Methods of education and evaluation	Wide and varied.	Same as school model but must be adapted to a widely heterogeneous group of learners; important to avoid "schoolishness" since many experience it as a deterrent to motivation.
Evaluative purpose	Criterion and normative (relationship to performance of other learners).	Almost entirely criterion (relationship to a standard of behavior).
Educational environment	Conceived as primarily educational but criticized as limited. Control is usually planned into the environment.	Commonly not conceived to be educational in purpose. Usually largely uncontrolled. Quite experiential in style.

the professional doing patient education occurs because the patient education model is so vague on this matter. Without a clear idea of the patient education model, many health professionals fall into a middle-class, professional-school-oriented model that assumes the prior development and necessity of basic learning skills such as reading, writing, and abstract problem solving. The health care system does not see its task as developing basic learning skills, but it clearly has to deal with people who do not have those skills. The outcome in the past has been a labeling of such persons as uneducable in health matters, largely from the standpoint of the middle-class, professional-school model. Now that that position is becoming no longer viable, the gradual move is to accommodate teaching materials and approaches to those with fewer skills. There are some patients who cannot profit from the altered approaches, who need at least minimal development of basic skills first. Such a combination of school education and patient education resources is, to say the least, not common.

3. Mediation of societal interests through physicians. Unlike the school, where societal interests are directly felt through the mechanism of lay boards and public votes for funds, patient education is still basically under the control of physicians. Only a very naive health care worker makes the mistake of forgetting this more than once. What he learns is a series of strategies to get around or incorporate the physician's concerns with patient education. There is disagreement on whether physician dominance of patient education ought to continue.

DEVELOPMENT OF A BROADER EDUCATIONAL MODEL

There is available a body of thought about universal principles of learning and teaching. The educative functions of some institutions, such as the family and the church, have been widely explored, although still with a considerable amount unknown about how they function. Other institutions, such as the health care system, have remained relatively unexplored and unconnected to the larger body of educational thought.

As Cremin suggests, schools of education have been essentially schools and departments of schooling. A modern school of education ought to look at education comprehensively and this means across the life span, and in all situations and institutions in which it occurs.[2] Such a development would be beneficial in many ways. The educative function of the health care system could be better understood, as could the interactions of its functions and the educative aspects of other institutions. For example, we now know only some of the ways in which the family mediates what the health care system teaches. The tasks for some patients are very difficult. The study of these tasks could be most informative in the development of basic theoretical knowledge about education.

SUMMARY

The school model and the patient education model are different and distinct, and mistakes can be made by confusing the two or when the patient education model is incomplete. An overall perspective of the educative functions of many institutions has been missing but promises to be significantly useful.

REFERENCES

1. Becker, M. H. The health belief model and personal health behavior. *Health Education Monographs,* 1974, *2(4)*, 409–419.
2. Cremin, L. A. *Public education.* New York: Basic Books, 1976.
3. Somers, A. R. (Ed.). *Promoting health consumer education and national policy.* Germantown, Md: Aspen Systems Corporation, 1976.

3

DEFINITION OF DESIRED BEHAVIORAL CHANGES

Behavioral changes that patients need to accomplish in the realm of health and illness are legion. A present health behavior may be defined as inadequate by the patient himself or by others, and he is faced with making a change.

There always has been a range of implicit standards about health action an individual or group should take. In addition, although still not generally accepted, the idea of the individual's responsibility to live in such a way that his health will be preserved is gaining support.[7]

Whatever the behavioral change, there is generally some agreement on the part of the patient and the system that the projected change is desirable. Specific changes are defined in the specialized books in this series. This chapter will focus on the problems in definition and acceptance of desired patient behavior changes.

CONCEPTUAL FRAMEWORKS FOR DEFINITION OF BEHAVIORS

Behavioral changes required by illness, for prevention of illness, or for promotion of health can be specific and precise procedures or can be major and induce changed self-concepts. Individuals differ greatly in the amount of assistance they need in making the behavioral change. Some change by themselves over a prolonged period, and it is not always easy to predict who will be successful.

This author believes that a major error in the way patient education is delivered today is its frequent orientation to learning knowledge or skills without placing these in the context of the patient as a person. While rehabilitation programs have commonly used a philosophy that deals with life in total, rehabilitation is used only in more profound disturbances such as damage to a spinal cord. The vast majority of patient education programs for those with chronic illness or learning a normal developmental task can be very specific and narrow.

ROLE DEVELOPMENT

Several such broad frameworks are available, one being role development. Transformations and developmental stages in health and illness directly initiate a number of important role changes. Education assists the patient to do some significant task or make a series of decisions that alter his situation or ability to play a role. For example, at the New Life Center at Family Hospital in Milwaukee, education is used to help provide control to the family, to give them a base for making decisions so that they can create the kind of childbirth experience they want.[17] The concepts of role insufficiency and role supplementation are a useful basis for nursing assessment and intervention. Modeling and role rehearsal are strategies to develop role clarity and skills.[13]

POSITIVE ADAPTATION

Concepts that describe a process of positive adaptation also are useful, such as a child's reestablishment of his body image after a disfiguring injury.[16] Teaching can also assist with a healthy resolution of a process such as the birth experience. One study found that many women could not completely reconstruct their childbirth experiences and became "stuck" on certain events they could not remember from their labor or delivery. They thought often about what they could not remember and sometimes were unable to focus on the present situation with the new baby. Long or rapid labors, high-risk conditions, or unfulfilled expectations seemed to make women more vulnerable to having "missing pieces" in their childbirth experiences. These women need to be helped with the reconstruction and understanding by someone who was there or who can provide factual data. Prescribed answers and dismissal of the patient's questions are not useful.[1]

On a broader level, anyone adapting to serious or chronic conditions searches for the meaning of the situation, attempts to ascertain the causes contributing to it, and to compare themselves with others. Clinical staff can play important roles in avoiding maladaptive responses resulting from the patient's fears, distorted meanings, lack of information, and failure to perceive viable alternatives.[12] Such patterns of response are useful ways to view the totality of teaching efforts. The effects of various parts of the teaching program then can be seen in the perspective of a whole response.

NURSING PRACTICE FRAMEWORK

A nursing practice framework also is of assistance, since it allows conceptual separation of the teaching done by nurses from that done by other health professionals and provides the goal for the practice. An example of this has been reported by Lucille Kinlein.[5] For her, nursing is assisting the person in his health care practices; teaching is an important intervention within this framework.

PREVENTING NEGATIVE EFFECTS FROM HEALTH INFORMATION

Finally, the educational function to yield understanding has been seen as critical to certain areas of care such as genetic screening, which inevitably raise anxieties in those screened. It is recommended that such screening be carried out under controlled conditions where education is effective and techniques for communicating are workable.[15]

These frameworks direct one toward a more complete intervention, one that is most likely to assist a patient in leading a healthy life.

MATCHING PATIENT'S AND THE SYSTEM'S DEFINITIONS OF BEHAVIORAL TASKS

The incongruence of the patient's goals and the system has been alleged many times and perhaps is inevitable. The incongruency can, however, represent political and social pressures to force behavior with a particular point of view. It can also represent a simplistic notion of the behavior to be obtained and the motivations that affect it, and can indicate learning or motivational problems on the part of the patient.

EXAMPLES OF MISMATCH

This kind of situation is described clearly in a study by Luker[11] of why women who were seeking abortions had failed to use contraception. The prevailing medical and, to a large degree, societal view is that any unwanted pregnancy should have been prevented or at least should have a history of attempts at prevention. There are two predominant professional views of why women do not use contraception: (1) they lack the contraceptive expertise to prevent pregnancies and (2) they have the expertise but encounter psychological resistance to using it (the psychoanalytic view).

The patient's perspective in making decisions about contraception (although not always conscious to her) is that she tries to attain many goals, only one of which is not getting pregnant, and includes commitment of the man involved. In addition, it is difficult for her to translate an 80 percent chance of pregnancy over the long run (from unprotected intercourse) into being 80 percent pregnant or estimate the likelihood of pregnancy to her from a specific act of intercourse.

She takes a cost-benefit approach to contraceptive use and at some time engages in risk taking, just as it is common in other areas of life to take risks with one's health: such as the decision to smoke or not to wear seat belts when riding in or driving a car. The cost of continued vigilant contraception includes: acknowledging being available for and engaging in intercourse, in some cases losing spontaneity; conforming to rules of the system for obtaining contraceptives; having a clear notion about whose responsibility (in a relationship) contraception is; and so forth. Women then weigh the actual cost of contraception (which they are experiencing) against a discounted risk of pregnancy. In addition, some event in their lives (such as imminent termination of the full-time mother role or death of a significant other) may change their evaluation of pregnancy, or they are tired of the contraceptive hassle and responsibility, which then sets the stage for risk taking.

The relevance of these findings for patient education should be addressed, even as one is clear that they may represent the experience and motivational patterns of only a portion of all women. Lack of expertise in contraception (as traditionally defined) is still a problem for some women. One could surmise that an additional kind of expertise useful for women would be conscious understanding of the differences between their models and those of health care systems, of how risk taking occurs and when it is likely, and of what actions can be taken regarding it.

Another example of mismatch of perspectives occurs when patients do not clearly differentiate the "purely physical" from the psychosocial, and the information they provide to clinicians is a product of both. Indeed, inability to differentiate symptoms of psychological distress from those of illness itself is common. Many illnesses, as well as medications for them, result in feelings comparable to those characteristic of high levels of stress or psychopathology. Fatigue, restlessness, and poor appetite, for example, may result either from depression or from an acute infectious illness.[12] Differentiation is a real problem.

Sometimes mismatches occur because societal norms do not encourage the educational program to be effective. For example, many studies have found venereal disease education not to be effective in prevention. Many of the traditional educational programs have centered learning basically on the factual or cognitive domain, with detailed study of the pathology (causative organism, mode of transmission, manifestation, diagnosis, treatment) of syphilis and gonorrhea. This approach might well be viewed as more appropriate for medical professionals and as irrelevant to the educational goal with teenagers. A goal stressed by present education is sexual abstinence; an implied goal is ability to remember signs and symptoms of sexually transmitted diseases, which are not simple even for physicians.[18]

An approach more congruent with norms of students (and hence one would predict more effective) would acknowledge that young adults will be sexually active and stress individual responsibility. Goals of such education would include being critical in choice of sexual partners, using preventive measures, accepting the possibility of contracting a sexually transmitted disease, and accepting responsibility to secure medical care if a person suspects infection.[18] Although still clearly not universally attainable, such goals represent less of a mismatch of instructional goals with the end behavior desired.

GENERAL APPROACH TO DEALING WITH MISMATCHES[6]

The differences in conception between patients and health care providers may be seen as the difference in models as, for example, the physician focusing on the disease while the patient focuses on the difficulty in living resulting from the disease. Patient–physician interactions can then be seen as transactions between explanatory models, often involving major discrepancies in cognitive content as well as in therapeutic values, expectations, and goals.

Patient models and popular explanations generally deal with one or more of the same five issues as described in the clinician's model:

1. Etiology
2. Onset of symptoms
3. Pathophysiology
4. Course of illness (whether acute or chronic, and severity of disorder)
5. Treatment

In general, patient explanatory models usually are not fully articulated, tend to be less abstract, may be inconsistent and even self-contradictory, and may be based on erroneous evaluation of evidence. Nonetheless, they are comparable to clinical models. Patient and family explanatory models may also differ.

Comparison of the patient model with the health care-giver's model enables the clinician to identify major discrepancies that may cause problems for clinical management. Such comparisons also help the clinician to know which aspects of his explanatory model need clearer exposition to patients (and families) and what sort of patient education is most appropriate. Often, the conflicts are related not only to different levels of knowledge but also to different values and interests. Clinical process involves negotiation between these explanatory models, once they have been made explicit.

Clinicians need to be trained to elicit the patient's model with a few simple, direct questions, and to formulate and communicate their model in terms that the patients can understand and that explicitly deal with the five clinical issues of chief concern listed previously. Models should be compared openly in order to identify contradictions and conceptual differences and to help the patient and care-giver enter into a negotiation toward shared models, especially as these relate to expectations and therapeutic goals.

Patients often hesitate to disclose their models. The following are questions that can elicit patient notions regarding the five key questions in the model:

1. What do you think has caused your problem?
2. Why do you think it started when it did?
3. What do you think your sickness does to you? How does it work?
4. How severe is your sickness? Will it have a long or a short course?
5. What kind of treatment do you think you should receive?

Some additional questions will elicit the patient's therapeutic goals and the psychosocial and cultural meaning of his illness, if these issues have not already been incorporated into his answers:

6. What are the most important results you hope to receive from this?
7. What are the chief problems your sickness has caused for you?
8. What do you fear most about your sickness?

An additional strategy used in another study was to explore the adequacy of preoperative teaching with postoperative patients who have undergone open heart surgery. This study clearly found need for specific information about the endotracheal tube, the mechanical respirator, mucus and suctioning, deep breathing and coughing, and chest tube removal.[14] While these findings are specific to the patient group studied, the approach can identify missing and poor instruction from the patient's point of view.

LENGTH OF MAINTENANCE OF BEHAVIOR CHANGE

In order to make an impact on health, it is felt that some basic behaviors need to be changed for a lifetime. The results of work in stopping smoking and reducing hypertension have also shown that people rarely maintain these initial changes over a long period of time. The factors that influence a patient to adopt a new behavior are not necessarily the same as those required to maintain it over time. Smoking cessation provides an example. A variety of techniques has developed that help smokers to stop smoking for a short period, but they show a remarkably high consistency in relapse rates.[19]

One option, of course, is a search for a very potent method of behavior change that will last. It seems more likely, however, that the sensitive, consistent, and thoughtful application of many reasonable techniques over a period of time is the strategy most likely to work. Elements that seem to make a difference in successful long-term change include health care systems that are responsive to individual needs over an extended period of time. This often involves a strategy of "titrating" the treatment program against the patient's response to the unavoidable difficulties associated with sustaining changes in life-style. This could include clarifying the problems through patient self-observation often reported in a diary, allowing the patient's past performance to set the next goal, assuring the patient that if he continues to try many different strategies over time his problems can be solved, and that the clinician is willing to support his efforts as he continues to try to make recommended changes. It is, in addition, important to tackle problems in progress soon after they occur rather than letting the patient experience a long period of failure and frustration.[19]

Short-term training influences are usually no match for the multitude of factors that affect a person's behavior in weeks, months, or years to come. Some care-givers arrange for continued patient contact after training but usually for purposes of assessment rather than a continuing effort to maintain initial changes.[19] It appears that special emphasis should be placed on recognizing the need for teaching intervention to assist maintenance of behavior change as a goal.

SELF-HELP AS A BEHAVIORAL GOAL

While it is clear that most (perhaps 75 percent) health matters have been dealt with by self-care, there is new interest in legitimizing and improving the quality of that care. This includes both continuous behaviors such as life-style, and episodic ones such as self-diagnosis and self-treatment. This interest has come predominantly in the United States from those who believe that all functions of health professionals are open to challenge and review for their potential transfer to the lay domain. People should develop a feeling of self-control and self-determination to act on their own priorities and to determine their own combination of risk. Appropriate and sound self-care has also been seen by the public and the system as a potential source of cost containment. The necessary skills must meet the demands of personal and community health, especially when many health problems must be solved by social action in the community.[8,9]

The general quality of most self-care is not known. A systematic review of studies has been done for self-help therapy manuals currently available. Programs for weight reduction, test anxiety, fear reduction, and exercise appear to produce at least short-term benefits, although some therapist assistance may be needed with weight reduction, and problems with subject follow-through often exist. A good deal of controlled research on smoking cessation has failed to identify a treatment program that produces lasting effects. Extensive validation is needed before treatment manuals for sexual dysfunction, assertiveness training, and child behavior problems can be used with confidence. Self-help programs are beginning to appear for problem-drinking, insomnia, and relaxation training but have not yet been validated. In general, the relevant and effective components of current instructional programs have not been identified.[3]

Perhaps the most distinctive element of the self-care approach, however, is its philosophical position. It runs directly counter to what may be the prevalant practice of the educator defining those learner concerns that are legitimate and appropriate, and of the expectation that the patient is to adapt to the system (compliance and cooperation as goals). Self-care builds on current lay health practices and supplements them with technical medical concepts, strategies, and skills not previously in the domain of family remedies. This is opposed to the more common approach of starting with the medical concepts and practices. The self-care approach would also suggest an analysis of the care-giver contributions to patient disability in the form of dependency-evoking activity, in an effort to have the total institutional environment contributing to patient growth in self-sufficiency.[10]

ETHICAL DECISIONS: CHOICE OF GOALS AND MEANS TO MEET THEM

There is a large number of ethical decisions in the practice of patient education because it involves transfer of information and power and skills from the care-giver to the patient. And because the accountability is operational in such a narrow part of the domain of patient education—primarily informed consent for medical procedures and care—there are many aspects of daily practice for which one feels a lack of ethical guidelines. Many of these questions can be characterized as concerning what learning goals for patients should be and if indeed there should be any.

The basic decision of whether to withhold information is guided generally by a decision by the physician of whether the patient would suffer great harm in knowing. There are wide disparities of opinion about effects on patients of knowing or not knowing their condition and little research to back either position. Neither is there much information about the realm of matters wherein having information is useful.

Additionally troublesome is the appropriate degree of directiveness of the patient educator/counselor in areas in which patients have had the right to make a decision. Genetic counseling and subsequent reproductive decisions represent such an area. Significantly, there is a broad spectrum of opinion among medical geneticists as to the nature and the limits of their obligations. Some believe the duty of genetic counseling is to provide estimates of risks (being a neutral educator), after which it is up to the couple to make up their own minds in light of the information given.[2] Genetics, however, is a field that is often difficult for lay people to understand, even after instruction. In addition, the present orientation of the field is to put the interests of the patient and family before those of society.[2] While this approach is characteristic of medical practice, it does leave unanswered ethical questions about society's interests.

An additional ethical decision concerns priority in making education available, given the limited resources that exist. An example based on criteria of cost-benefit potential and the present level of effectiveness with such behaviors may be seen in Figure 3-1. It represents essentially a public health approach that clearly conflicts with what some individual patients need. As might be expected, neither the public health nor the individual patient welfare approach adequately describes how decisions on priority are made, which is usually on political bases and on grounds of custom.

If a decision is made to change a patient's behavior, the professional has a responsibility to use the appropriate treatment modality, i.e., one that is the most effective and efficient and also the least intrusive. Of considerable importance is predicting and monitoring negative side effects of the teaching intervention (see Chap. 8).

Points of view about client ethical responsibility are being more widely heard today. These especially focus on potentially damaging behaviors such as smoking with the question of why society through insurance, welfare and veteran's benefits, etc., should pay for the individual's self-inflicted damage.[7] Such responsibility may be more widely required in areas that are truly under the patient's control; addictive behaviors may perhaps be viewed differently.

SUMMARY

The area of definition of desired behavioral changes in patients is filled with conflict and lack of clarity, perhaps reflecting the basic ambivalence surround-

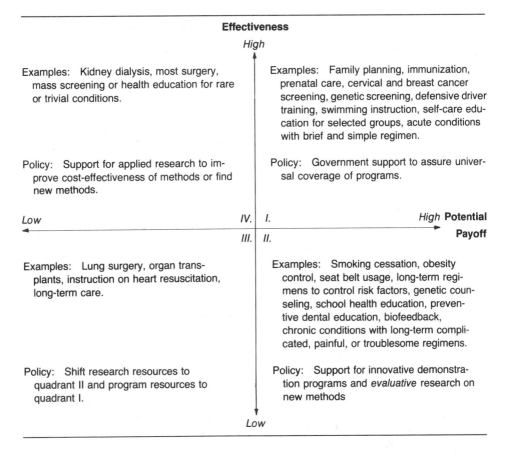

Effectiveness

High

Examples: Kidney dialysis, most surgery, mass screening or health education for rare or trivial conditions.

Examples: Family planning, immunization, prenatal care, cervical and breast cancer screening, genetic screening, defensive driver training, swimming instruction, self-care education for selected groups, acute conditions with brief and simple regimen.

Policy: Support for applied research to improve cost-effectiveness of methods or find new methods.

Policy: Government support to assure universal coverage of programs.

Low   IV. | I.   *High* **Potential**

III. | II.   **Payoff**

Examples: Lung surgery, organ transplants, instruction on heart resuscitation, long-term care.

Examples: Smoking cessation, obesity control, seat belt usage, long-term regimens to control risk factors, genetic counseling, school health education, preventive dental education, biofeedback, chronic conditions with long-term complicated, painful, or troublesome regimens.

Policy: Shift research resources to quadrant II and program resources to quadrant I.

Policy: Support for innovative demonstration programs and *evaluative* research on new methods

Low

FIGURE 3-1.
Policy implications for health strategies classified according to effectiveness and cost-benefit potential. (Adapted from Green, L. *Determining the impact and effectiveness of health education as it relates to federal policy.* USDHEW Contract Sa-7974-75, 1975, p. 51.)

ing patient education. Flexible use of broad patient-oriented conceptual frameworks is uncommon, and mismatches between patients' desires and those of the system are not unusual. Indeed, some whole areas of care, such as long-term maintenance of behavior change, have been neglected although they are clearly required for patients to reach goals that society generally supports. As might be expected, forums for discussion and resolution of the identifiable issues are rare.

REFERENCES

1. Affonso, D. E. Missing pieces—a study of post-partum feelings. *Birth and the family,* 1977, *4,* 159–164.
2. Cowie, V. A. Genetic counseling clinics, in Raine, D. N. (Ed.). *Medical-social management of inherited metabolic diseases.* Lancaster, England: MTP Press, 1977.

3. Glasgow, R. E., & Rosen, G. M. Behavior biblio therapy: A review of self-help therapy manuals. *Psychological Bulletin,* 1978, *85,* 1–23.

4. Green, L. *Determining the impact and effectiveness of health education as it relates to federal policy.* USDHEW Contract SA-7974-75, 1975.

5. Kinlein, M. L. A self-care concept. *American Journal of Nursing,* 1977, *77,* 598–601.

6. Kleinman, A., Eisenberg, L., & Good, B. Culture, illness and care: Clinical lessons from anthropologic and cross cultural research. *Annals of Internal Medicine,* 1978, *88,* 251–258.

7. Knowles, J. H. Responsibility for health. *Science,* 1977, *198,* 4322.

8. Levin, L. S. The lay person as the primary health care practitioner. *Public Health Reports,* 1976, *91,* 206–209.

9. Levin, L. S., Katz, Alfred H., & Hoist, E. *Self-care: Lay initiatives in health.* New York: Prodist, 1976.

10. Levin, L. S. Patient education and self-care: How do they differ? *Nursing Outlook,* 1978, *16,* 170–175.

11. Luker, K. *Taking chances: Abortion and the decision not to contracept.* Berkeley: Univ California Press, 1975.

12. Mechanic, D. Illness behavior, social adaptation and the management of illness. *Journal of Nervous and Mental Disorders,* 1977, *168,* 79–87.

13. Meleis, A. I. Role insufficiency and role supplementation: A conceptual framework. *Nursing Research,* 1975, *24,* 164–170.

14. Miller, S. P., & Shada, E. A. Preoperative information and recovery of open-heart surgery patients. *Heart and Lung,* 1978 *7,* 486–493.

15. National Academy of Sciences. *Genetic screening programs, principles and research.* Washington D.C.: National Academy of Sciences, 1975.

16. Smith, E., Livskie, S., Nelson, K., & McNemar, A. Reestablishing a child's body image. *American Journal of Nursing,* 1977, *77,* 445–447.

17. Timberlake, B. The new life center. *American Journal of Nursing,* 1975, *75,* 1456–1461.

18. Yarber, W. New directions in venereal disease education. *The Family Coordinator* 1978, *27,* 121–126.

19. Zifferblatt, S., & Wilbur, C. S. Maintaining a healthy heart: guidelines for a feasible goal. *Preventive Medicine,* 1977, *6,* 514–525.

4
MANAGING PATIENT LEARNING

Teaching is the use of a set of intervention strategies to create learning (see Chap. 7 for differentiation from other kinds of psychosocial strategies). That this service is offered as part of a professional practice implies that the professional has special skills and will obtain more positive outcomes than will a lay person. This means that he knows how to manage learning, including use of directive intervention when necessary.

The simplest and most common way to conceptualize teaching strategies is as an interaction among a learner, an environment, and a teacher, more or less directed by the teacher. In general, the strategies used are interpersonal between teacher and learner or between learner and other persons in the environment, written and pictorial materials, and observation and practice of performance. The learner's thinking is a very major focus of teaching interventions since thinking mediates most actions.

Management of learning requires knowledge of and ability to use the patient's abilities, which differ widely. Since more specific information about population subgroups will be provided in other books in this series, only a few examples will be given here.

People's thinking abilities vary considerably, based on their age, physiologic and psychosocial health, learned ability, and so forth. For this reason, when teaching an aged adult whose thinking ability is somewhat impaired, one might (1) select a place and time when simultaneous activity in the environment will be minimal in order that competing stimuli will not disrupt the person's learning; and (2) integrate new behaviors with established and ongoing behaviors so as to enhance memory.[12]

It is well known that teaching approaches to children must be adapted to their developmental stages. For example, the preschooler unquestioningly accepts his own perceptions; questions help him to express his rationales and perceptions, which are then amenable to correction. He also often needs help in understanding that there are impersonal reasons for illness and procedures that divest them of their moral and punitive overtones, i.e., "It's something I did wrong." Since his first symbols are nonverbal, his absorption and recall of information is enhanced when one does not rely solely on words but also provides him with visual, auditory, tactile, and motor images.[22]

Similarly, teaching of patients with strokes requires adaptation to their deficits. One nurse found left hemiplegics often distracted by peripheral sounds such as television and so taught them in a quiet training room. Right hemiplegics have difficulty understanding or responding to instructions and so require slow talking, giving them time to assimilate and respond, and the use of gestures and demonstrations.[15]

Some areas of health education have existed as a part of a social movement, not thoroughly integrated with the health care system. They often have their own traditions and definitions of purpose, content, method, and philosophy. Some of these movements, even though they have existed for a long time, frequently have used a variety of teaching approaches, often with a very thin base of empirical support for their practices.

An example is the field of parent education. Its activities were estimated to have begun in this country in the early 1800s, becoming more formal in the 1920s and 1930s. A variety of professionals and nonprofessionals teach in parent education programs under the auspices of mental health, schools, and other associations, using every imaginable form of media. Parent education has been aimed primarily at middle-class parents with young children. Content often includes child development, general personality functioning, child-rearing techniques, methods of discipline, emotions and their expression, interpersonal communication, parent–child relationships, and so forth. The methods used have been adopted from the disciplines of counseling, psychotherapy, and education with the approach adopted tending to follow the leader's theoretical beliefs about how children should develop. There is no universally agreed upon method in parent education. It uses primarily group methods, with individual approaches having become more identified with family or child therapy. Training of parents in behavior modification techniques is recent, and, because it has occurred to help parents deal with individual specific behavior problems, has been considered therapy. What research there is commonly fails to show differences in theoretical points of view and has not tested results over extended periods of time. A present focal point in parent education today is advocacy of more democratic methods of child rearing often identified as the Dreikers-Adlerian Approach and the Gordon Approach using Parent Effectiveness Training.[7]

These general definitions and an example of the social structure in which some education exists form a backdrop for some common concerns in managing education. These include basic decisions about structure and detail of content and learning activities, obtaining and prolonging retention, use of the context of learning, and making learning opportunities available. Some practice follows more purely one particular theoretical point of view; some of these are presented. However, much practice uses an eclectic blending of these points of view, perhaps drawing most heavily on the one that best seems to explain the situation in which one is working.

RETENTION OF LEARNING

The quality of initial learning is important for long-term retention. A structure for meaning will often be remembered long after detail is forgotten and will be an assist for the reconstruction of learning. Strong initial learning to the point of mastery or overlearning is also useful for prolonging retention. This makes all the more worrisome the unplanned, intermittent, brief approach to patient education which is not uncharacteristic in some settings. Such an approach can mean that thorough learning is never accomplished. An example of a teaching program that aims to attain mastery is that described for clean self-catheterization of the urinary bladder by children. As soon as catheterization is mastered in one position, the child is assisted in performing the procedure in other positions such as his wheelchair, sitting on the toilet, and standing. He learns the procedure with and without braces. He is given the opportunity to do the catheterization in a variety of settings and positions and is assisted with adaptations that are necessary at home and in school.[1]

Breaking a task into parts and mastering each part in sequence is a way to assist complete learning. Some people will only half-learn a complex skill without this approach. For example, steps in taking a pulse may be feeling it, noting its rhythmicity, and then counting it.

Making important statements specific rather than general can assist patients in recalling them. For example, very soon after an interview with a physician, patients are unable to recall a high proportion of what they have been told, and instructions or advice are even less well remembered than are diagnostic statements. The perceived importance of a medical statement has been shown to be directly related to the likelihood of its recall. More specific statements ("Take two full weeks holiday a year") are seen as more important than those formulated in general rules[4] ("You need frequent holidays").

Both mental and physical rehearsal can serve to periodically strengthen learning that would be forgotten through disuse. The patient can prompt himself to do this or can be prompted by someone else such as the nurse at his regular clinic visit.

One of the most difficult aspects of patient education as presently practiced is its limitations of timing and setting. If given, patient education is commonly delivered when the patient is receiving physical or medical treatment, often in a hospital or clinic. This means that he is often trying to learn about situations he has not yet experienced, and it also means that corrective feedback from a teacher commonly is not available when he tries his skills at work or at home "for real."

It seems as if exceptionally slow progress is being made in getting health education delivered more adequately. Before better patterns of delivery are widely developed, there will probably need to be some resolution of issues of cost-benefit of patient education and of reimbursement for it. In the absence of services more ideally delivered to support learning, realistic simulation would be an assist. The patient is given multiple opportunities to practice in a situation like the one in which he will be functioning. At present, such simulation is not widespread and is seen as more important for complex medical procedures such as home hemodialysis than for other learning, especially when the patient will be returning home to a remote area. The simulation in this instance may involve the patient and his family living in a home and managing the dialysis themselves.

STRUCTURE

Structuring refers to limiting and organizing the elements of the learning situation in order to assist the patient in his efforts to change his behavior. Structuring can be done both to the content to be learned and to learning practice. Many health-rela ›d situations are experienced by patients as complex and ambiguous; they have high emotional loading and can be interpreted in many possible ways. This makes them confusing and formidable.

Structure can be simple, like a daily drug reminder chart developed to improve patient compliance. One study showed that use of such a chart with name of drug, dosage, use, and time(s) of administration explained by the pharmacist significantly increased compliance in comparison with a group who had only the pharmacist's explanation.[8] The presence of the chart serves as a reminder, and it gives the basic information necessary to take the drug.

Contracting with patients provides a structure for the entire teaching interaction. It commonly sets goals and time frame, describes roles and process, and indicates conditions for renegotiation of the contract. It does not usually address the structure of the content. Its strength is in the clarity it adds to the process of teaching-learning and the mutual commitment implied in the signing.

Follow-up or supervision programs often provide a structure for expectations and reinforcements. This can be done by telephone or as part of a more elaborate system of follow-up visits to the home as part of an outpatient care program.

The health professional has to structure the teaching tasks. The necessity of teaching patients about a wide variety of topics requires more spontaneous competence than many nurses feel they have. For this reason, protocols such as the one in Table 4-1 have been developed.

ELABORATION AND DETAIL

While structure provides a framework that organizes content and process, there still remains a teaching decision about the amount of detail it is wise to ask the patient to learn. Ideally, this decision should be based on empirical evidence, studies that indicate the amount of information necessary for many patients to take adequate health actions. In the absence of this research base, one makes the decision about elaboration on other grounds, such as patient interest, the teacher's notion of proper amount of detail, and so forth.

A large amount of detail can often be comprehended if there is a structure or device on which to "hang" it, that is, something that links learning elements in a web of meaning. An analogy is such a structure, and it is often useful to introduce it before training to establish a context as well as to return to it during training. Conditions in which key relationships are complex and not visible lend themselves to analogies. One example is the explanation of the

TABLE 4-1.
PROTOCOL FOR TEACHING HYPERTENSIVE PATIENTS

Education About Blood Pressure
Step 1.   Assess patient's knowledge by asking if he knows the normal levels of blood pressure and the meaning of systolic and diastolic readings.
  a. If yes, proceed to *Step 3*.
  b. If no, proceed to *Step 2*.
Step 2.   Provide information, using visual aids as available.
  a. Define blood pressure as the amount of pressure that blood exerts on the inside walls of the arteries.
  b. Define systolic blood pressure as the
    • highest pressure in arteries when the heart is pumping or contracting
    • first sound or thump heard when taking a blood pressure
    • top number in the recorded blood pressure measurement, and as
    • normally below 140 mm Hg.
  c. Define diastolic blood pressure as the
    • lowest pressure in arteries when heart is relaxed or filling
    • last sound or thump heard when taking a blood pressure
    • bottom number in the recorded blood pressure measurement, and as
    • normally below 90 mm Hg.
Step 3.   Obtain feedback.
  a. Ask patient to state in his own words:
    • the meaning of blood pressure
    • the difference between systolic and diastolic pressure
  b. Show patient printed recordings of normal and abnormal systolic and diastolic pressures.
  c. Ask him to identify systolic and diastolic pressures and to say if they are normal or abnormal.
Step 4.   Apply knowledge, using sphygmomanometer, blood pressure cuff, and stethoscope.
  a. Take patient's blood pressure, but do not tell him the readings.
  b. Retake patient's blood pressure, letting him use the stethoscope to listen to his blood pressure sounds. (Nurse controls release of cuff pressure unless patient already knows how to do this.)
  c. Tell patient to record his blood pressure measurement.
  d. Evaluate accuracy of the recorded readings. Praise the patient if correct. If incorrect, repeat b and c.
  e. Ask patient to say whether his readings are within the normal or abnormal range.
  f. Ask patient to state upper limits of normal systolic and diastolic blood pressure.
Step 5.   Correct misinformation. Explain any errors or gaps in knowledge as indicated by patient's responses to e and f. Repeat *Step 2* if indicated.

Education About Hypertension
Step 6.   Assess patient's perceptions and feelings by asking
    • what having hypertension means to him in terms of his health and life-style
    • what he thinks might have caused his hypertension
    • what he has been told about hypertension by others
Step 7.   Discuss perceptions and feelings by
    • correcting any misinformation about hypertension
    • discussing any fears related to having hypertension
    • discussing any guilt feelings related to the patient's development of hypertension

(*continued*)

TABLE 4-1
PROTOCOL FOR TEACHING HYPERTENSIVE PATIENTS (Cont.)

Step 8.   Assess patient's knowledge by asking him to tell what he already knows about hypertension in regard to the following (omit items already discussed in *Steps 6* and *7*): definition of hypertension, cause, risk factors, basic pathology, symptoms, long-term complications, and changes in life-style to control hypertension.

Step 9.   Provide information (omit items discussed in *Step 8*).
  a. Define hypertension as repeated blood pressure readings in the adult higher than 140/90 mm Hg.
  b. Explain that hypertension and high blood pressure mean the same thing; hypertension does not mean that a person is high-strung or nervous; specific cause is not known in 90–95% of people, and therefore the condition is called primary or essential hypertension.
  c. Define a risk factor as something that makes a person more likely to develop hypertension. The risk factors for hypertension are: family history of hypertension and/or heart disease, obesity, diabetes mellitus, increasing age, chronic heavy sodium intake, and being a black male.
  d. Help patient identify his risk factors.
  e. Describe the basic pathology as a narrowing of the small arteries that increases the pressure in them and makes it difficult for the heart to pump blood through them. Eventually arteries become weak and burst or become so narrow that blood cannot pass through them.
  f. Explain that symptoms often are not present, but damage still occurs. If symptoms are present, they do not indicate how high the blood pressure is.
  g. Discuss long-term complications of uncontrolled hypertension: damage to the heart, brain, kidneys, and eyes (sometimes called target or end-organ damage). Arteries in target organs become weaker and/or narrower so that blood has difficulty flowing through, and the heart is overworked and becomes larger and weaker.
  h. Mention the changes in life-style that are important to control hypertension: achieving ideal body weight; restricting sodium intake; exercising daily for at least 30 minutes; learning techniques to relax and reduce stress in daily life; not smoking; not using drugs which elevate blood pressure—cold tablets, nasal sprays, estrogen hormones, pep pills, diet pills; continuing to have blood pressure monitored periodically even if not being followed regularly for drug therapy; and keeping appointments for follow-up care if on medication.

Step 10.   Obtain feedback by asking patient to state in his own words what he knows about the items explained in *Step 9.*

Step 11.   Correct any errors or gaps in knowledge. Repeat information from *Step 9* as indicated.

Step 12.   Answer questions and ask if there is anything else about hypertension that patient wants to know or discuss.

Step 13.   Establish the contract.
  a. Help patient and family (if present) decide what specific changes in life-style are needed to help control the patient's blood pressure.
  b. Help patient decide the amount of change he will strive for.
  c. Record specific life-style changes that have been agreed to.
  d. Give patient a copy of the contract.

Step 14.   Arrange for return visit, to evaluate progress, including time to discuss in more detail the problems of altering life-style.

From Mitchell, E. S. Protocol for teaching hypertensive patients. *American Journal of Nursing,* 1977, 808–809. Copyright 1977, American Journal of Nursing Company. Reproduced with permission from *American Journal of Nursing.*

action of insulin in diabetes. One analogy used to explain this topic was "as a mailman carries a package to your mailbox, so insulin carries sugar to the cell."[13] But the teacher should be careful; analogies often also include elements that can lead to misinterpretation. It is wise to anticipate those elements and point them out to patients.

Similar difficulty with conceptual learning and necessity for use of an analogy was found in a program for teaching clinic patients the rationale for their peptic ulcer regimen. It was found impossible to teach neutralization of acid to the patients, who had no adequate concept of acids, and it was necessary to understand not only acid but neutralization, secretion, and hypersecretion. (Hypersecretion was taught with the use of the analogy of a dripping faucet.) Learning about ulcers was slow partly because patients commonly held misconceptions that were incompatible with the material being taught. For example, the misconception that antacid coats the stomach was extremely persistent until the point was made that antacids do not coat the inside of the mouth (which is like the stomach) although they do coat the lips (which are unlike the stomach).[6] This study of patients with ulcer found that the conceptual approach which was being tried was effective primarily in patients with average intelligence or better. It was concluded that the instructor should identify the more common contingencies and provide specific instructions for dealing with them, rather than relying exclusively on comprehension.[6]

Additional instructional elements become important, depending on the character of the behavior to be attained.

FREQUENCY[10]

If a health action must recur periodically and the goal of the program is to establish a pattern of regularity, then health education methods which provide cues at appropriate intervals tend to be more effective than one-shot or sporadic methods. For example, telephone or mail reminders can improve appropriate frequency of prenatal visits, annual pap smears, dental visits, and other such periodic tests.

Consider frequency of action for immunization: Adults need act every 10 years, whereas children need many doses, especially in the preschool years. Therefore, the educational approach should be different from that aimed at frequent activities, such as eating, exercising, or taking medication. It may be beneficial to encourage a regular source of care, to encourage personal record keeping, to educate at strategic times, and to build reminder systems into institutions such as schools and workplaces that already keep health records.[26]

PERSISTENCE[10]

If the required health behavior is one that must be continued over a long period, as with medical regimens for hypertension or diabetes, then reassessment and reteaching and provision of social supports in clinic and home environment improve effectiveness.

RANGE OF BEHAVIORS AND DISTANCE TO TASK[10]

In some situations, such as rehabilitation counseling and education of parents of disabled children, a large number of behaviors must be learned. Sometimes, also, desired behaviors require considerable change from past behaviors, usually in changing of living style, e.g., diet, recreation, work, family relationships, exercise, doing a treatment regimen. An example is the patient with renal failure who will be on home dialysis. These situations require longer and more intensive instruction, often in multiple settings, and teaching and reinforcement of graduated steps are included in the behavioral repertoire.

All of the above elements in the desired behavior must be determined in order to properly design the instructional treatment. This kind of analysis assists one in making decisions about the amount of elaboration and detail necessary.

AVAILABILITY OF INSTRUCTION

For a person who cannot learn by himself, a basic need is access to instruction. With a wide range of learning abilities, the amount of time spent learning is highly predictive of the outcome.[3] Also critical is the quality of the instruction, including the availability of accurate feedback to correct mistakes and reward good performance. Some experts believe that time may be a more useful way of determining normal human variation in learning than the notion of inborn ability, especially as individuals are brought to a fixed criterion of attainment.

The evidence about availability of instructional opportunities in health care settings is slim. There is very little information about the variety of opportunities individual patients have to learn. Descriptions of specific formal programs of patient education are more commonly reported. Results of such a survey show formal programs of patient education concentrated in certain topics. For hospital-based patient education, these are hypertension, diabetes, and nutrition; for Health Maintenance Organizations (HMO), weight control, prenatal care, hypertension, diabetes, smoking and how to use the system; for public health departments, short-term, nonintensive teaching regarding child care and nutrition education for young parents, education on health services and resources, and on common public health problems such as drugs, venereal diseases, lead screening, and dental health.[19]

That the instructional opportunities are sometimes limited is clear. Consider this description from a study that found inner-city parents had significantly less information regarding common health care for children than suburban parents. The inner-city pediatrician almost never knew the mother and baby from the newborn period, since his patient turnover rate might be 50 percent or more each year. He frequently saw the family in a noisy and hurried setting. The family often had received conflicting advice from a series of other doctors.[25]

Self-help clubs have many reasons for existing and probably would exist even if health education were improved. At present, the movement is neither strong enough nor large enough to reach more than a fraction of the population in need. But these clubs assist with incorporating social processes into the dynamics of coping and adjusting to the rehabilitative requirements of chronic illness, which is said to be poorly done by the health care system.[11] The consumer position about health education is that it should be available for purchase and that much of it need not be controlled by the physician.

KNOWLEDGE ABOUT THE EFFECTS OF CONTENT

Determining what content to teach a patient is not as obvious as it may seem, especially if one wants a behavioral outcome in which motivation or control of emotion plays an important part. The prime example is compliance with a health regimen—a knowledgeable patient who gets supervision and support does not necessarily comply. In general, the clinician simply uses his best judgment about the content the patient can tolerate and needs to solve his problem.

Knowledge about content is just beginning to be available. Probably the best established (through research studies) content approach to distressing health procedures is that studied with adults and children undergoing invasive and stress-producing procedures such as a gastroendoscopic examination or children having an orthopedic cast removed. Consistently, this research has shown that individuals who are given no preparatory information and those given only procedural information, that is, explanations of how and where the procedure will be done, experience greater distress than do those who have been told what is felt, tasted, heard, seen, and smelled during the event. This transcript is an example of providing sensory information.

Hi, I am a nurse. I would like to tell you what it is like to have your cast taken off. First you will hear the buzz of the saw like this (pause, followed by the sound of the saw). The doctor will use the saw to cut two sides of the cast. He will cut only as far down as the padding over your skin. The saw will not cut you but you will feel vibrations or tingling when the cast is cut. And you will see chalky dust flying around. It may also feel just a little warm. None of this will hurt and it certainly won't burn you. You will feel vibrations or tingling and warmth and will see chalky dust.

Next the doctor will remove the padding and you won't feel anything then. Your skin under the padding will be scaly and will look dirty because it has not been washed for a long time. Your arm or leg may be a little stiff when you first try to move it and your arm or leg may seem light because the cast was heavy.

I have told you what it is like to have your cast taken off, now remember what will happen: you will hear the buzz of the saw, see the dust, and feel warmth and vibrations or tingling when the cast is cut off.[16]

POINTS OF VIEW ABOUT LEARNING

Scientific evidence about human learning does not support any one grand comprehensive theory. Rather, work has been done on various points of view, each of which yields some evidence that can be used in understanding learning. Several of these approaches are summarized here.

ADULT LEARNING AND DEVELOPMENT[17,18]

This point of view focuses on the strategies for adult learning and the changes that come with advancing age. Adults can be assisted to learn when:

1. they have a chance to be self-directed in setting learning expectations, pace, and preferred learning resources.
2. a structure of the content and process of learning are provided and when links are made between organized knowledge and personal experience, current competence and new learning.
3. the greater task orientation of adulthood, especially around life problems, and problem solving as a way of thinking is capitalized on.

Learning change in older adults and ways to help them compensate include:

1. providing memory aids to help with the decline in short-term memory capacity.
2. providing sets of categories and other structures to help with increased difficulty organizing complex material.
3. minimizing distracting and irrelevant information activities to help with more difficulty discarding irrelevant aspects in learning situations.

BEHAVIOR MODIFICATION[9]

Behavior modification is not only a mode of therapy but also a way of understanding individuals, of focusing on the interaction between the environment and the individual, and includes both internal and external events. This approach draws from social learning theory. In the account which follows, the practical aspects of this body of thought are emphasized.

Assessment involves identification of the events that cause and maintain behavior. The emphasis is on observable, countable responses, such as frequency, magnitude, or duration of behavior, and thought or feeling. Internal dialogue consists of what a person anticipates is going to happen, how he interprets the past, and how he evaluates his behavior and that of others. Distortions in his thinking may include taking something for granted, blowing an event out of proportion, and overgeneralization; intervention involves altering misconceptions. A patient may not know how to behave, or the behavior not be reinforced by, for example, group or cultural norms. Determining why the behavior does not occur can be established by role playing, and then the behavior may be taught or reinforcements established, depending on which is appropriate. Since both thoughts and feelings can result from a change in behavior, assessment of the patient's problem involves a decision about whether certain thoughts should be a major focus for intervention.

An example of use of behavior modification is development of self-management skills in regulating stress. These skills are particularly useful when it is not possible to locate the source of anxiety or anger, and general skills are needed because stress occurs in a variety of situations. Such procedures train the client to discriminate antecedents of stress—his cognitions and feelings and sensory awareness of physiological cues—and to use these as cues to utilize certain reactions. The assessment should reveal which response systems are particularly involved, such as the affective, cognitive, or behavioral, and focus the intervention accordingly. The stress inoculation program used with multiphobic clients aims to educate the client (formation of a mutual conceptualization of anxiety) about the nature of stress reactions, to have the client rehearse coping skills, and to offer the client opportunities to practice coping behaviors in which anxiety is experienced and successfully reduced.

BIOFEEDBACK[5]

The emphasis in biofeedback is on body responses to emotion and to mental processes and their use to alter subtle body activity such as muscle tension or heart rate. The patient uses different kinds of information to create these physiological changes. Biological information is given by the biofeedback signal. The therapist provides information about what the physiological activity does, how it behaves, and how it is measured; clues for changing physiological activity by "mental means"; and psychologically supporting information, which is encouragement and reinforcement that serves to consolidate the learning experience. Experiential information which is internally derived information from association of the biofeedback signal with internally perceived changes in mind and body states is learned by the patient.

MEMORY[20]

Basic information about how memory may best be understood to function can be used to enhance retention of material important to the learner. Information first enters through one of the sense organs and is stored very briefly, usually within a second or so. Some of this information is transferred into the next store, which is called short-term store.

Short-term store has a limited capacity; it can hold seven plus or minus two chunks of information. A chunk is anything that has some unitary representation like a single number or like a proverb. A single unfamiliar telephone number may represent about as many chunks as short-term store can hold. A person is vastly able to improve his short-term store capacity by judiciously recording many low-information chunks into fewer high-information chunks. Information in short-term store is in general lost within about 15 seconds unless it is placed in a special section of short-term store called a rehearsal buffer. By rehearsal, repeating it over and over again, the information does not decay.

The final component of this system is long-term store which is the virtually unlimited capacity store of that information that we have more or less permanently available to us. Our ability to speak a language is an example of something in the long-term store. Information is presumably transferred into the long-term store from the short-term store. This occurs by memorization.

Retrieval involves transferring information from long-term to short-term store, although the retrieval may include only part of the information needed.

Assistance for reducing memory loss comes basically through organization and rehearsal and by not overloading the system's capacity. Organization aims at making more comprehensive chunks and can be done with categories, stories, or with imagery. A patient can be helped to relate material into chunks that make sense to him and that do not interfere with (are not too close in meaning to) other information he has learned. Rehearsal can be done by prompting oneself to recall the information or by someone else doing so. Overload can occur by having too many unrelated chunks of information without enough time to deposit them in the long-term memory.

Sometimes forgetting is caused by temporary retrieval failure. A different situation provides the right retrieval cue and the information becomes accessible, i.e., remembered. Development of memory cues is important in patient education. The cue should be in the environment in which the patient will be carrying out the behavior and be a cue he knows will trigger the particular memory organization structure.

THE CONTEXT OF LEARNING

There are many circumstances surrounding learning that appear to profoundly affect it through their reinforcing value, the clarification or confusion they cause in objectives, and by their ability to make instruction available or not. These circumstances include public attitudes and understanding about a particular health problem, the degree of integration of a staff and the model they follow in giving care, and the degree of available knowledge about cause and treatment of the health problem. Because these matters seem to be "just part of the situation," they may well not be identified as affecting the range of learning options and the success of teaching.

In school, such contextual matters have been called the "hidden curriculum," which may or may not be congruent with the formal written curriculum. Health teaching often has a very strong "hidden" curriculum, which is in conformity with both medical concepts, and, by extension, conformity with the way that system operates and advice it gives. Examples of contextual elements in health teaching follow.

GENETIC COUNSELING

This area suffers from very abstract concepts, for which there often is not an adequate knowledge base either in the lay public or among health professionals. In addition, social guidelines for behaviors are both lacking and in a very rapid state of transition. For most individuals who participate in the genetic screening process, the disease for which they are being screened is an unknown and abstract entity, as for example in Tay-Sachs disease. Furthermore, they are not being tested for disorders that they themselves may acquire or that would affect their personal health, but for what is known as a predisposition that could affect their future offspring. Other complex information that must be given includes the definition of being a carrier, prevention of personal and ethnic stigmatization, severity and prognosis of the disorder, the notion that risks exist only when two carriers produce a child, estimation of what those risks are for each pregnancy, and knowledge of availability of prenatal diagnosis and prevention. This complex information must be targeted to the community prior to screening without creating hysteria.[23]

In addition, there is evidence that neither the medical profession as a whole[24] nor the public has what might be called an appropriate level of knowledge about genetic disease. This has the effect of not providing social support for becoming knowledgeable in the area. It also means that instructional opportunity is not readily available directly from physicians. These are two powerful contextual variables.

STUDY OF PARTICULAR REHABILITATION AND NEPHROLOGY UNITS

A study by Hill[14] which compared perceptions of clients and personnel about the rehabilitation process is an example of a number of studies which try to describe interactional dynamics on units and eventually link those dynamics to patient outcome. The messages which were transmitted and the restraints on communication form at least part of the context for learning for patients.

In the physical rehabilitation units studied, there was little clarity of roles and little input from clients or nurses regarding the rehabilitation process. Clients were highly religious and because the medical model on which the unit was operating was never explained to them, they had difficulty seeing the relevance of the requirements placed on them in the unit.

On the nephrology unit, the staff perceived clients from a limited acute medical perspective rather than as being rehabilitated. The patients were told of their disabilities, but they were not provided with the second step of the rehabilitation model, which is not only establishing capacity but utilizing capacity.

OTHER FACTORS

These include the certainty of diagnosis, progression, and prognosis; the degree of disruption caused by a disease process and treatment of it including the difficulty of a self-administered treatment; and whether the treatment produces any positive effects. Persons who have long-term chronic disabilities or illnesses often make strenuous attempts to see their medical history as a whole, to connect together everything that has happened to them in an attempt to provide a coherent story. In one such group of persons, those who were the most satisfied with the information they had received were those who had undergone surgery. A possible reason for this is that the operation provides a structure for the information-giving procedure; preoperatively the patient is told what is to be done and postoperatively there is further explanation. In the long drawn-out course of a complex illness such a focal point may never be reached.[2]

SUMMARY

Management of learning uses knowledge about learning and the contexts in which positive experiences for it are available to support the patient's efforts to change his behavior. Decisions about structure, content, and detail, and about use of the environment are made with the goal being for the patient to achieve as much learning as possible and to retain it during a certain period of time or under the necessary circumstances.

REFERENCES

1. Altshuler, A., Meyer, J. & Butz, M. K. J. Even children can learn to do clean self-catheterization. *American Journal of Nursing,* 1977, *77,* 97–101.
2. Blaxter, M. *The meaning of disability: A sociological study of impairment.* London: Heinemann Educational Books, 1976.
3. Bloom, B. S. Time and learning. *American Psychologist,* 1974, *29,* 682–688.
4. Bradshaw, P. W., Ley, P., Kincey, J., & Bradshaw, J. Recall of medical advice: comprehensibility and specificity. *British Journal of Social and Clinical Psychology,* 1975, *14,* 55-62.
5. Brown, B. B. *Stress and the art of biofeedback.* New York: Harper, 1977.
6. Caron, H. S., & Roth, H. P. An evaluation of a program for teaching clinical pa-

tients the rationale of their peptic ulcer regimen. *Health Education Monographs,* 1977, *5(1),* 25–49.

7. Croake, J. W., & Glover, K. E. A history and evaluation of parent education. *The Family Coordinator,* 1977, *26,* 151–158.

8. Gabriel, M., Gagnon, J., & Bryan, C. Improved patient compliance through use of a daily drug reminder chart. *American Journal of Public Health,* 1977, *67,* 968–969.

9. Gambrill, E. D. *Behavior modification: Handbook of assessment, intervention and evaluation.* San Francisco: Jossey-Bass, 1977.

10. Green, I. W. *Determining the impact and effectiveness of health education as it relates to federal policy.* USDHEW Contract SA-7974-75, 1976.

11. Gussow, Z., & Tracy, G. S. The role of self-help clubs and adaptation to chronic illness and disability. *Social Science and Medicine,* 1976, *10,* 407–414. *Journal of the American Dietetic Association,* 1975, *66*:465–470.

12. Hallburg, J. C. The teaching of aged adults. *Journal of Gerontological Nursing,* 1976, *2(3),* 13–19.

13. Hassell, J., & Medved, E. Group audiovisual instruction for patients with diabetes. *Journal of the American Dietetic Association,* 1975, *66*:465–470.

14. Hill, C. E. Differential perception of the rehabilitation process: a comparison of client and personnel incongruity in two categories of chronic illness. *Social Science and Medicine,* 1978, *12,* 57-63.

15. Huston, J. C. Overcoming a learning disability of stroke. *Nursing,* 1975, *1,* 66–68.

16. Johnson, J., Kirchoff, K. T., & Endress, M. P. Easing children's fright during health care procedures. *MCN,* 1976, *1,* 206–210.

17. Knowles, M. *The adult learner: A neglected species.* Houston: Goff, 1973.

18. Knox, A. B. *Adult development and learning.* San Francisco: Jossey-Bass, 1977.

19. Little AD Inc. *Executive summary: A survey of consumer health education programs.* DHEW Contract 100-75-0082, 1976.

20. Loftus, J. R., & Loftus, E. R. *Human memory: The processing of information.* Hillsdale, N. J.: Lawrence Earlbaum, 1976.

21. Mitchell, E. S. Protocol for teaching hypertensive patients. *American Journal of Nursing,* 1977, *77,* 808–809.

22. Pidgeon, V. A. Characteristics of children's thinking and implications for health teaching. *Maternal-child Nursing Journal,* 1977, *6(1),* 1–8.

23. Rimion, D. L., Greenwald, S., Nathan T., & Kaback, M. Unique consideration for genetic counselling in community based carrier screening programs, in Kaback, M. (Ed.). *Tay-Sachs disease: screening and prevention.* New York: Liss, 1977.

24. Rosenstock, I. M. Public health aspects of Tay-Sachs screening, in Kaback, M. (Ed.) *Tay-Sachs disease: screening and prevention.* New York: Liss, 1977.

25. Tomlinson, W. A. Parents' knowledge of respiratory disease: a comparison of inner-city and suburban parents. *Pediatrics,* 1975, *56,* 1009–1013.

26. Yokan, C., & D'Onofrio, C. Application of health education methods to achieve higher immunization rates. *Public Health Reports,* 1978, *93,* 211–215.

5

SUPPORTING PATIENT MOTIVATION

Simply stated, motivation deals with why people do things. But motivation is apparently very complex and poorly understood, affected by events in the environment as well as by a person's needs and his general ability to direct himself. Motivation consists of general directions as well as some very specific ones relative to a particular temporal situation.

Behavioral theory stresses reinforcement as motivating (such as attention or relief of symptoms); cognitive theory stresses needs and interests. People have different reasons for engaging in the same behavior. It is common for multiple motives to operate simultaneously in any individual, and motivation changes from time to time. One study of adherence to a medical regimen for control of hypertension illustrates the complexity of the interrelationships among variables that might motivate a patient to comply. For example, social support might not lead to adherence by itself, but it might encourage a patient who felt competent to meet the demands of the regimen to take the first step. The link between the demands of the regimen and its perceived interference was likely to be strongest when the patient had many competing motives.[4]

When a change in behavior is required, the most trouble-free situation is likely to occur with a person who:

1. is intrinsically motivated (wants to feel competent and is self-determining in dealing with his environment)
2. is mastering the tasks of his developmental stage and the tasks of adaptation to his illness
3. has beliefs regarding health that are congruent with those of the care-giver and who has a fairly high knowledge level in that belief system.
4. has an environment that can be supportive in attaining and maintaining the new behavior, thus creating natural ongoing rewards for that behavior.

Others will likely have additional barriers to changing their behavior.

LIFE TASKS AND PROCESSES OF ADAPTATION TO ILLNESS AS MOTIVATIONAL CONTEXTS

Life tasks and disruption of them by disease can create a motivational stage for specific learning. An example can be seen in end-stage renal disease. A person in the middle years who is on dialysis may well have no tools with which to compensate for his loss of youth. He has lost the energy with which to compete in the job market. He may be apprehensive about the loss of family love, and he may not have the means to change his life or to keep it the same if he wishes to. He has to be dependent at a time in life when persons become independent.[9]

Children who have long chronic illness may have arrested development and may become passive and dependent. Young children have difficulty in coping with the immobility required during dialysis. They have poorly developed abstraction skills and so are subject to misinformation and may think they are being exsanguinated. The child's developing defenses are poorly structured and easily subject to disruption leading to regression. Neither children nor adolescents communicate their conflicts well.[3] This background is likely to affect the tasks the patient sets for himself, including whether he feels it is worthwhile to comply with medical care.

In addition to a stage of development in life tasks, patients and families are also locatable in stages of adaptation to a health problem or in readiness to take a health action. Table 5-1 describes a model of psychological adaptation to hemodialysis. While in its general phases the model is not unlike that for adaptation to other diseases or to grieving, each health problem does present specific psychologic concerns. A program aimed at forestalling untoward reactions of spouses to patients' beginning and adapting to dialysis was not successful, probably because it did not fit the stage of adaptation of the clients. The massive use of denial and the anxious worry, pity, and sympathy on the part of the significant other rendered both of them poor candidates for a psychoprophylactic intervention. Some months later (during postdialysis I or II) may be an excellent time to have group meetings for emotional ventilation, mutual support, reinstituting socialization behaviors of both persons, and so forth.[10]

BELIEF SYSTEMS

Every cultural group has a system of beliefs about health and illness, with an internal logic that governs its continuous borrowing of concepts. These systems may well yield different points of motivation. For example, one system lumps all kinds of illness and specifies neither particular ones nor specific causes; others have extensive classification systems. Someone from the "lumping" system has no motivation (sees no reason) for further specification. More specific conflicts in health beliefs with scientific medicine are described by Snow,[12] who studied popular medicine in a black neighborhood. Humoral pathology beliefs

TABLE 5-1.
A MODEL OF THE PSYCHOLOGY OF ADAPTATION TO HEMODIALYSIS
FROM DIAGNOSIS TO LONG-TERM ADJUSTMENT

Predialysis: Renal Failure Dialysis From Diagnosis of End-Stage to the Begining of Regular Dialysis		Postdialysis I: Beginning to 4-6 Months of Dialysis		Postdialysis II: The Long-term Adjustment from 6 to 12 Months of Dialysis	
Patient	*Significant Other*	*Patient*	*Significant Other*	*Patient*	*Significant Other*
Massive use of denial (sometimes maintained with the hope of transplantation).	Denial used but less than patient.	Moderate denial focused at medical prognosis.	Slight use of denial.	Resolves grief process; tolerance for one's fate; "resignation".	Often shows exceptional involvement in kidney-related groups, or minimization of patient's disabilities.
Preoccupied with maintaining premorbid functioning.	Worries about patient, suppression of own feelings; minimizes implications ESRD has for altering own life-style.	Resents own fate, struggles to integrate limitations into self.	Resents fate of patient with beginning awareness of own altered life-style.		
Intense anxiety over unknown.	Anxious over fate of patient.	Anger at "normality" of staff, physicians, and friends.	Anger at staff, physicians, and friends for failure to ameliorate the problems.	Anger mainly in reaction to reality-based limitations.	Capable of getting angry at patient; may act out anger by withdrawal, separation, divorce; anger at friends and family whc have terminated social contact.

Sometimes clinically depressed.	Depressive feelings.	Depressed.	Depressive feelings.	Chronic, low-grade depression.	Periodically depressive feelings.
Because of denial, anxiety, and worry, remains ignorant of details of dialysis and in that sense is ignorant.*	Denial, anxiety, and worry result in poor learning of details, although usually not to the extent of the patient; sometimes compulsive following of physician's orders.	Withdrawal behaviorally and emotionally.	Confused and bewildered by loss of social contact.	Concern about sexual dysfunction.	Worry about sex.
		Self-pity. (Why me?)	Self-pity.		
Uremic.	Massive sympathy for patient.	Overdependent.†	Overwhelmed with reality problems, often confused and helpless; a "needy" person.	Overdependence on others stabilizes into chronic semidependent pattern.‡	
				Sadness over significant other's life-style changes.	Fear of death of patient.

*Are a few exceptions who "flee into facts" and are excellent learners.
†Although sometimes counterdependent.
‡Occasionally a fierce independence occurs.
From Newton, J.R. Psychoeducational meetings with the spouses of ESRD patients. *Dialysis and Transplantation*, 1978, 634. Reproduced with permission.

are still prevalent in this group, especially focused on blood. Blood is believed to go "up," "down," is "thick" or "thin," "high" or "low," and so on, and is most prominently affected by diet. So a woman diagnosed as having a light stroke felt that her blood had "boiled up" giving her "blood in the brain." She was sitting up in bed since she felt this would allow the blood to drain back down. She had thrown away the medicine prescribed by a physician who said that she would always have to take it (conflicts with the notion that every malady has a cure).

Probably the major model that predicts readiness and motivation to take action in the health field today is the *health belief model*. It indicates that a health action is not likely to be taken unless the person has the following four beliefs about it:

1. He believes himself susceptible to the disease in question.
2. He believes the disease would have serious consequences if he should contract it.
3. He knows how to reduce the threat, which is treatment.
4. He believes that the threat of the treatment is not as great as that of the disease.

Generally, a cue is necessary to trigger an action.[1]

This model has been used with a variety of disease entities and preventive care and, while not uniformly highly predictive, is by far the best tool we have today. It can be used as an initial screening tool to see whether the patient has the beliefs necessary to take a health action, or it can be used to focus intervention into inducing the beliefs that seem necessary.

An example of use of the *health belief model* is the production and use of a film on birth control education, specifically focused at sexually active adolescents. National surveys have found that about one-half of this group failed to use any kind of contraception the last time they had intercourse. One of the most significant attitudes in this group (at least as found by some surveys) is the belief that one could not become pregnant. Sometimes adolescents believed that they were too young, that they had sex too infrequently, or that they had intercourse at the wrong time of the month. There may be lack of factual knowledge of birth control, but these questions may also indicate guilt over sexual behavior and subsequent refusal on the part of some girls to acknowledge that they are having intercourse. Translated to the *health belief model,* this is a deficit in belief #1. Related is a difficulty with belief #4 since another reason that has been found for nonuse of birth control is the fear of seeing a physician, of purchasing contraceptives at a pharmacy, or of being discovered by parents.

A film was then developed to try to address the common patterns and beliefs found in this group of teenagers. The film included personal discussions with young women who had experienced pregnancy including a group of pregnant adolescents, a girl who gave up her child for adoption, and a girl who had an abortion. The discussion centered on the reasons why these young people did not use birth control during their sexual relations. This strategy is obviously aimed at belief #2, which is clarifying the seriousness of not taking the health action, and at belief #1, by using highly credible subjects, with whom the audience could identify, telling their rationales.[8]

PATIENT MISCONCEPTIONS AS MOTIVATING INFORMATION

Analysis of misconceptions of patients and families illustrates the natural attribution of meaning in a foreign situation and the need for instruction. Of course, such analysis does not examine all the times in which patients' conceptions (often learned informally) are correct. But some misconceptions can form a critical link in the patient's thought patterns and lead to unwarranted conclusions and motivations. They are often common to a particular group of patients and can be anticipated.

Some misconceptions are common because bodily sensations cannot be counted on to differentiate conditions. One such misconception is that angina mimics a heart attack. Other forms of information to which the patient does not commonly have access, such as the electrocardiograph, provide verifying data. A similar misconception has been found among blue-collar patients, who knew nothing about scar formation and pictured their hearts as permanently punctured.[6] This image, and the belief that another heart attack would occur, could well be critical misconceptions.

Care-givers may be able to do a better job than they have been in avoiding critical misconceptions. Less adequate communication between health-care givers and patients from lower-class backgrounds has been documented consistently. One-half the blue-collar patients interviewed in one study interpreted artifacts as coming from their hearts rather than from the monitors. Such misconceptions can create much unnecessary stress.[7]

SUPPORT OF THE ENVIRONMENT

Environmental support is necessary both to initiate and to maintain the learning process. High anxiety is not unusual in health teaching since patients are often dealing with the threat of, or actual loss of, a significant aspect of health. In such a situation, the patient can easily be overwhelmed and give up on learning. He can be assisted to continue with memory support, easy and concrete tasks, clear directions, and teacher feedback about what he is doing. Sometimes changing the situation by redefining the task or by modification of the social interactions is helpful, and sometimes gaining the skills that a patient thinks he needs takes the pressure off.

Supportive health environments allow easy access to information, including being available at times when the patient feels the need for information, having easy access to personnel as in getting appointments, and having efficient operations (not long waiting times) so as not to inconvenience the patient.

Social support in the lay environment includes assistance with tasks, consultation, continued social interaction, understanding of the patient's health needs, and helping him carry them out. Such support is often seen as an essential element for long-term behavior change.

POSSIBLE INTERVENTION STRATEGIES TO SUPPORT MOTIVATION

In order to support motivation, the teacher can manipulate

1. the task (difficulty, abstractness, length)
2. the learner's perceptions (about difficulty of the task and how he is doing)
3. his relationship with the learner
4. the reward structure

For example, theoretical knowledge indicates that persons with a strong need to achieve do better with goals of intermediate difficulty; persons with a strong need to avoid failure prefer very easy goals. The teacher can assist motivation by helping the patient set goals of the proper level of difficulty. Clinical examples follow.

Perhaps one of the simplest strategies may be negotiation between health care-giver and patient, that is, if the parties view their relationship that way. The strategy accepts the fact that the patient and care-giver may well have different and conflicting goals. The parties involved should state their goals and then seek to understand the points at which these goals converge. Negotiation involves each party making his point, with each listening to the other's point and then responding.[2] This pattern helps to make certain that each understands the other and then assists with commitment by the kind of compromise goal that results from the negotiation. This approach primarily manipulates the relationship with the care-giver.

Another approach to motivation is to help the patient develop skills and support that can avoid feelings of hopelessness. Such an approach has been outlined for patients with chronic obstructive pulmonary disease, a condition for which there is no treatment known to reverse or even stop its progression. Development of social supports, coping ability (ability to change the environment to meet one's needs), and adaptive ability (ability to adapt oneself to the existing environment) are believed by some to motivate the patient and his family to avoid chronic disorganizing emotions that can upset or destroy the therapeutic program.[11] This approach addresses both the definition of the task and the learner's perceptions.

Some patients with end-stage renal disease, including those learning home dialysis, reach a state called oversaturation during the learning process. The

Health Belief System	
Present knowledge of hypertension:	
perceived causation	—attributes elevated blood pressure to being overweight and stress at work and home
perceived severity of own hypertension	—does not consider present BP level serious; thinks it would require medication if it remained in the high 90 range (diastolic)
feelings about length of therapy	—doesn't like to think about taking medications for an indefinite length of time
perceived efficacy of regimen	—concerned about the "safety" of medication; "maybe someone will discover they cause cancer three years from now. . . ."
Significant others' past experience with BP meds	—none
family awareness and concern for treatment	—wife occasionally checks both of their blood pressures; hers is generally higher than his; she does not think she needs medication, either
Implications of being on medication:	
degree of anxiety when first diagnosed	—surprised, but not overly concerned
impact of having hypertension on life	—states "taking pills would remind me that I am sick, but I feel well"; rarely absent from work due to illness
Feelings about health issues:	
rating of health among life priorities	—job and family concerns more important than his own health at present, especially since he feels well
importance of BP control in relation to other risk factors/ health problems	—interested in monitoring BP; not concerned about present cholesterol (too hard to change); plans to stop smoking someday
feelings of control in health matters	—feels able to control BP with weight loss
in other situations	—(work) states his job is handling problems and he is pretty good at it
	—(personal life) there have always been problems at home, but they always seem to work themselves out without asking for outside help
interest in participating in "self-care" activities	—not interested in learning home blood pressure monitoring himself, but does weigh himself every day at home
Past experience with the health care system/providers	
positive _____	—experience has always been "illness oriented"
negative _____	
none _____	

Figure 5-1.
Hypertension assessment form: portion about health belief system. (From Foster, S., and Kousch, D. C. Promoting patient adherence. *American Journal of Nursing,* 1978, *78,* 829–32. Copyright 1978, American Journal of Nursing Company. Reproduced with permission from *American Journal of Nursing* .)

Name: __Mr. R.G.__

Date: __12/12/77__

Record Number: __000-000__

Session Objective:

1. __Evaluate the need for medication__

2. __Assess progress in weight loss program__

3. __Discuss modifications of other risk factors__

4. _____

Present Antihypertensive Regimen: none

Visit Data BP Reading # 1 __132/94__   goal DBP ____86____ mm Hg

BP Reading # 2 __128/92__   1.2 × ideal weight   180   lbs.

BP Reading # 3 __130/93__   current weight ____188____ lbs.

Strategies

BP Value:

feedback   [X]   Discussed the feasibility of beginning medications today,

reinforcement   [ ]   since DBP remains above 90 mg Hg; Mr. G. agreed

Medication Regimen:

adherence assessment   [ ]   ┌──────────────────────────────┐
reinforcement   [ ]   └──────────────────────────────┘

adherence strategies:

pill taking schedules   [ ]   —will take medication in A.M. when he brushes his teeth;
"cues"   [X]   keeps meds in medicine cabinet

report of side effects [ ]   —Close friend recently died from a heart attack; wife's recent
obtaining medications   [ ]   hospitalization made him start to think about his own health

discussion of health   —home blood pressure readings taken by wife were lower
beliefs   [X]   than clinic readings (taken nightly for a week)

home blood pressure
monitoring   [X]   —CONTRACT: CALL CLINIC BEFORE STOPPING PILLS
"contracts"   [X]   OR IF INTOLERABLE SIDE EFFECT DEVELOPS

(continued)

Figure 5-2.
Portion of hypertension encounter form. (From Foster, S., & Kousch, D. C. Promoting patient adherence. *American Journal of Nursing*, 1978, *78*, 630–631. Copyright 1978, American Journal of Nursing Company. Reproduced with permission from *American Journal of Nursing*.)

Understanding the Regimen:

Name, dose, frequency	[X]	—may need to periodically adjust the dose and type of medi-
Action	[X]	cation needed
Precautions	[ ]	—diuretic "water pill"; works by reducing the circulating
Common side effects	[X]	blood volume
Length of therapy	[ ]	—expect increase in urination and perhaps fatigue especially
		the first week of therapy

Appointment Keeping:

assess barriers	[ ]	
reinforcement	[ ]	
phone call communication	[ ]	

Nonpharmacologic
Interventions:

dietary

sodium intake	[X]	—has reduced the amount of table salt used; now tastes food
potassium intake	[ ]	before adding salt; discussed the use of other nonsodium
alcohol intake	[ ]	seasonings (lemon juice, herbs, powders vs salts)
weight loss	[X]	—has lost 7 lbs in the past two months; DPB still not
exercise	[ ]	below 90 mm Hg; emphasized continued slow weight loss
stress reduction	[X]	as *adjunct* to medication, to perhaps avoid the need for
smoking cessation	[X]	stronger medication
other	[ ]	—refused referral to Social Services or staff psychologist to
		discuss family problems
		—has set cigarette smoking *quit date of January 1st*

Instruction:

blood pressure physiology	[ ]	
etiology of hypertension	[X]	
consequences of untreated hypertension	[ ]	
control of hypertension	[X]	—expresses hope that some day he will not need medication
		to control BP
factors affecting blood pressure	[ ]	

FIGURE 5-2. (Cont.)

earliest symptoms are described as nonverbal, often vague somatic complaints, excessive dependency, a diminished response to instruction, an inability to reproduce what the patient has previously learned, and an increase in errors made by the patient. If his symptoms are not recognized, he may begin demanding that the materials be presented in a different manner, or that his instructor be changed, or he may show suspicion toward staff members. The staff may respond to these coping mechanisms by presenting more educational aspects, which in turn feed additional fear and anxiety. Verbal expressions of anger are described as coming at the point when the patient's tolerance for more learning is at an absolute minimum.[13]

These signs of oversaturation might well be interpreted as problems with the material being presented; a likely alternative explanation is the patient's difficulty in coping with the demands of his illness. In either case, motivation is disrupted. The suggested intervention is to back way from the learning process, let the patient know you are reading his frustrations, and be willing to listen. This intervention manipulates the nurse's relationship with the learner when the learner's perceptions become distorted.

Utilizing several of the theoretical approaches outlined above (*health belief model* and social support theory), two nurses[5] developed an educational assessment and counseling approach for helping patients with hypertension adhere to their medical regimens. The *health belief system* portion of their hypertension assessment form and the hypertension encounter forms are reproduced in Figures 5-1 and 5-2. The authors report that listing strategies in this manner on the encounter form helps to ensure that adherence-related interventions are performed consistently.

SUMMARY

Motivation in health situations is affected by emotional reactions, beliefs, understandings, and misconceptions. Environments supportive to making a behavior change, including the environment constructed for teaching, assist with motivation.

REFERENCES

1. Becker, M. H. The Health Belief Model and sick-role behavior. *Health Education Monographs,* 1974, *2,* 409–419.
2. Bernarde, M. A., & Meyerson, E. W. Patient-physician negotiation. *Journal of the American Medical Association,* 1978, *239,* 1413–1415.
3. Bernstein, D. M. Life with ESRD—children and adolescents. *Dialysis and Transplantation,* 1978, *7,* 424–428.
4. Caplan, R. D., Robinson, E. A. R., French, J. R. P., Caldwell, J. R., & Shinn, M. *Adhering to medical regimens: Pilot experiments in patient education and social support.* Ann Arbor: Institute for Social Research, The University of Michigan, 1976.

5. Foster, S., & Kousch, D. C. Promoting patient adherence. *American Journal of Nursing,* 1978, *78,* 829–832.

6. Hackett, T. P., & Cassem, N. H. *Coronary care patient psychology.* New York: American Heart Association, 1975.

7. Hackett, T. P., & Cassem, N. H. White collar and blue collar responses to heart attack. *Psychosomatic Research,* 1976, *20,* 85–95.

8. Herold, E. S. The production and use of an attitudinal film in birth control education. *Journal of School Health,* 1978, *48,* 307–310.

9. Landsman, M. Adjustment to dialysis: The middle years. *Dialysis and Transplantation,* 1978, *7,* 432–434.

10. Newton, J. R. Psychoeducational meetings with the spouses of ESRD patients. *Dialysis and Transplantation,* 1978, *7,* 632–637.

11. Rowlette, D. B., & Dudley, D. L. COPD: psychosocial and psychophysiological issues. *Psychosomatics,* 1978, *19,* 273–279.

12. Snow, L. Popular medicine in a black neighborhood, in Spicer, E. H. (Ed.). *Ethnic medicine in the southwest.* Tucson, Arizona: Univ Arizona Press, 1977.

13. Vrana, L. Patient learning: where is the saturation point? *Journal of the American Association of Nephrology Nurses and Technicians,* 1977, *4* (suppl. ed.) 50-51.

6

METHODS OF PATIENT INSTRUCTION

This chapter approaches instruction from several levels of generality, trying also to make clear conceptual links with the learning that it is hoped will result. Beginning with the broadest notion of general styles of teaching and learning, the chapter then moves to characteristics of instructional modes and the differences in stimuli and experiences they present. Particular approaches have been seen as useful for teaching motor skills and attitudes; the general teaching methods, having been originated in school learning, usually adequately present cognitive learning opportunities. Next, analysis is made of particular approaches as they have been applied in patient education. These are methods which resemble packages of general activities for teacher and learner. And finally, comments are made about how programs of patient education should be viewed as embodying large numbers of instructional decisions, which can be improved and reformulated if they are viewed as more than a series of unrelated instructional acts.

LEARNING AND TEACHING STYLES IN PATIENT EDUCATION

Patients reflect the range of general learning styles present in the public, but they may well operate in a less flexible mode than usual when under stress.

In reality, learning styles represent points on continuums. Some of these are the following:

1. Concrete versus abstract. Some persons learn best from actually visualizing and experiencing a task or an idea. Others, who have more verbal skills, can learn from symbols alone and then can perform.
2. Inductive versus deductive. Some persons learn best by learning rules and then deducing actions from those rules. Others learn by having experiences and, based on those, forming their own operating rules.
3. External versus internal locus of control. Some persons believe that fate controls their lives; others believe that they can greatly influence what happens to them by learning about it and using that knowledge.

Persons have different combinations of these and other learning styles; generally the style of those with less formal education is concrete, inductive, and external in locus of control. Formal education directly teaches abstract thinking and how to operate from rules, and gives a feeling of competency in influencing others. Certain subject matter or patient education tasks lend themselves to certain learning approaches. For example, early approaches to home hemodialysis training seem to have focused on understanding abstract ideas as well as learning skills. Diabetes education programs that lean toward complete understanding of the condition often are abstract with a strong focus on controlling one's fate. It is generally easier to accommodate the kinds of learning styles found in the highly educated since it is then possible to directly use approaches common in professional education.

There is a point of view that social class position affects personality development by providing differential learning experiences, which for any given class consist of its distinctive value system and interaction patterns. This would, of course, yield certain learning styles. The patterning of these values and themes is outlined in Table 6-1, with the work in this field summarized by Lundberg.[14]

Importantly, social class hierarchy is believed to represent a developmental hierarchy; that is, the model personality of the higher class represents a higher level of maturity. These characteristics include not being dominated by the immediate, concrete situation; having capacity for delay and planning; not being driven by one's own affective states; actively manipulating the environment; having an accurate perception of others' motivations; and an appreciation of the needs of others and of group goals. Social class may, then, be indicative of the kinds and diversity of learning supports already present, and of differences in world view between middle-class health professionals and persons of working and lower classes.

A key question is whether patient educators ought to try to adjust materials and approaches to the patient's natural learning style. An alternative, of course, is to indicate that there are certain prerequisite behaviors and learning abilities and that without these patients cannot be taught. In the future, health professionals had better be very sure of such statements, since such demands will be challenged.

GENERAL TEACHING STYLES

Since teaching activity provides opportunity for learning, teaching styles can be thought of on the same continuums as learning styles. For example, a person rated highly on external locus of control may well respond better to authoritative demands than to a logical, reasoned, high information approach that leaves motivation for the desired behavior dependent on the internal motivation of the patient.

TABLE 6-1.
THE PATTERNING OF SOCIAL CLASS VALUES OR THEMES

Middle-Class Values	Value-Dimension	Working-Class Values	Lower-Class Values	Value-Dimension
Active mastery Manipulation Open world-view; change, flux, movement	Activity	Striving for stability and security Belief in luck or fate	Powerlessness in impersonal and achievement areas	Passivity
Faith in rationalism Preference for orderliness	Rationalism	Traditionalism Attitudes held unquestioningly Pragmatism and antiintellectualism Oral and local tradition	Antiintellectualism and intolerance	Traditionalism
Universalistic ethic Stress on equality rather than hierarchy	Universalism	Person-centeredness Home and neighborhood centeredness The personal and the concrete	Simplification and narrow experience and perspectives	Particularism
Emphasis on individual personality	Individualism	Person-centeredness Home and neighborhood centeredness "Them" vs "us"	Deprivation Misanthropy	Primary group orientation
Strong orientation toward change and the future	Future orientation	Excitement The immediate, the present, the cheerful No point in saving Belief in luck or fate	Toughness Insecurity	Present orientation

From Lundberg, M.J. *The Incomplete Adult: Social Class Constraints on Personality Development.* Westport, Conn.: Greenwood Press, 1974, pp. 18,19. Reproduced with permission.

Teaching styles can be broadly characterized as fitting into general approaches which differ in their conceptions of what is to be learned as well as what activities support learning. Some examples are the following:

Academic Approach. This fits most closely with the school model of learning. Goals often include considerable understanding of the scientific aspects of the health condition in the hope of providing a valuable base for patient decision making and acceptance of the task. In terms of learning styles, this approach emphasizes the abstract, often working best with a person having strong internal control. Academic learning materials are often used, involving a great deal of reading and providing useful vicarious experience for the patient. Such an approach often assumes a high development of learning skills. It can be an expensive approach if it is carried out primarily with reading materials. However, its effectiveness in teaching patients to carry out actions may be lacking and may be erroneously assumed. Persons who have not been successful in school learning may not only be unable to learn from this approach, but may also have strong negative emotional reactions to it.

"Do It" Approach. In this approach, the ability to carry out actions is most highly valued, and learning activities focus on concrete demonstrations and practice. Learning "why" is not seen as being of great importance and certainly not as the major or only activity of learning.

Support Approach. The primary focus is support for the patient's natural ways of coping and achieving a health behavior. Reinforcement and emotional support from persons in environments in which the patient will be using the new behavior are seen as critical. Information and skills are given but often in an informal, unstructured interaction with the patient and his significant others, and triggered by what the patient indicates he needs and is ready to learn.

Matching teaching styles with the learner's style and the requirements of the subject matter or skill he is trying to learn probably produces the best results. Each health professional probably has a preferred style. At the extreme there are some patients who cannot learn from a strongly academic focus, and, if that is all that is being offered to them, it cannot be said that professional teaching service is being rendered. A health professional should be able to use several approaches, but, failing that, someone who can match his teaching style to the patient's learning style should be available.

INSTRUCTIONAL MODES

Instruction represents stimuli that assist with learning. Instructional modes have developed that differ in the learning stimuli that they provide: no one mode provides all stimuli (Table 6-2). Likewise, learning tasks differ, and so the key lies in choosing a mode that will present most of the conditions needed to accomplish the learning. For example, a person to undergo sex change surgery may need to learn social skills that are more appropriate to the new gender. Demonstrations, practice, and role-playing modes will be more useful since they provide practice of the new skills that the transsexual can use in real social situations. In discussion and lecture modes, such opportunities are rarely available and the focus on transfer is relatively weak.

In schools, many kinds of concept and verbal association learning are impor-

TABLE 6-2.
KINDS OF LEARNING OPPORTUNITIES IN VARIOUS INSTRUCTIONAL MODES

	Gains and Maintains Attention	Gains and Maintains Motivation	Provides for Immediate Feedback and Reinforcement	Provides for Practice	Provides for Organization	Allows Patient to Progress at Own Rate	Provides for Transfer
Lecture	Potentially	Potentially	No	No	Yes	No	Potentially
Discussion group	Usually	Usually	Usually	Potentially	Seldom	Potentially	Usually
Tutorial with nurse	Yes	Yes	Yes	Potentially	Potentially	Yes	Potentially
Demonstration/ practice	Usually	Potentially	Usually	Yes	Sometimes	Yes	Potentially
Role playing	Yes	Yes	Usually	Usually	Potentially	Potentially	Yes

Adapted from Shuell, T.J., and Lee, C.Z. *Learning and Instruction*. Monterey, Ca. Brooks/Cole, 1976, p. 139.

tant. Problem solving that a patient is motivated to do in an independent situation is probably the primary type of learning in patient education. The methods seen as excellent for teaching problem solving include discussion, tutorial, role playing, and projects (such as doing one's own care.) Lectures, recitation, and drill are good for the kind of learning done in schools, but rarely for problem solving.

So, because patient education is designed to increase patient skills rather than cognitive development, certain of the generally available methods of instruction are more useful than others. Methods that provide practice, lots of feedback, reinforcement, and correction, and those that require patient participation during learning are more likely to be successful. Lectures or materials that do not provide participation and feedback are not likely to be optimal for very many learners, especially when more than minor behavior changes are desired.

One method that would seem to have potential, but is rarely used at present, is the case study approach. Case studies are down-to-earth, attention-holding, experiential, and holistic, and can serve to increase conviction. Case studies are sometimes created by placing patients in contact with other patients who then serve as living examples. This could well be extended by using written case studies or describing them orally. One fear in using such an approach is that patients will overgeneralize or incorrectly generalize from the case example to their own situation. This difficulty can be decreased by choosing cases from which patients can correctly derive information. The fact that it is not a highly controlled teaching method (the patient is expected to draw some of his own conclusions) may cause reluctance regarding its use.

PATIENT PARTICIPATION AS A KEY INGREDIENT

Learner participation is a valuable goal for the process of instruction, since the quality of this participation is usually a good index of the quality of the learning that is occurring. Participation means that the patient is operationally a part of the decision about goals to be met, chooses a learning method and style, regularly demonstrates what has been learned to date, and helps to judge whether the learning is adequate for his needs.

Participation includes elements that assist in learning such as feedback and correction, reinforcement, practice, and so on, especially considering the dangers of the highly verbal, abstract learning styles that health professionals often unwittingly use with patients. Participation allows quick evaluation of the success of any learning materials used.

Remember that speed of initial learning is not related to quality of final learning. The more something is practiced, the better it is learned; the better it is learned, the better it will be remembered. Participation and active feedback and correction will keep the teaching-learning process on track and avoid the notion that if learning has not occurred in a certain period of time, it never will.

The kind of participation essential to teaching problem solving is critical to patient education. Problem solving must be based on the prior attainment and recall of rules basic to the problem at hand. As a method of learning, it requires that the learner discover a higher order rule, constructed in his own idiosyncratic way, himself. Instruction is supportive and can include guidance about ways to approach the problem but must finally allow the learner to do it himself. This creates a highly effective capability that generalizes to many situations and is highly resistant to forgetting.[6]

CLINICAL ROUTINE AS INSTRUCTION

We must constantly think of clinical acts and behavior requested of patients as instructional. One study, done with cirrhotic patients, who are often considered relatively unreliable and noncompliant, forms an illustration. These patients were asked to make daily telephone reports for 6 months on weight, alcohol ingestion, medication, general activity, hours worked, abdominal girth, and so on. Patients were highly cooperative. Apparently, the self-measurement routine was reinforcing to the patients, and use of feedback to them positively influenced to health habits.[7]

ON THE "EVILS" OF AN OVERLY VERBAL APPROACH

A highly verbal approach, especially written prose, is a predominant element of the school model that frequently is overused in patient education. It is effective and seems comfortable to many health professionals, but the major focus of patient education is not literacy. The major dangers of this approach, which is a form of instruction aimed at understanding scholarly knowledge, is that patients cannot translate it into reality, and it makes instruction inaccessible to those who do not have the skills to understand it. This does not mean they cannot learn, however.

In addition to its verbal character, such instruction often takes on the characteristics of scientific knowledge, which can be quite at variance with the patient's common sense. Common sense is more action oriented, more particular and concrete, socially conceived rather than logically conceived, and uses illustration and example rather than definition and deduction.[17] Verbal, scientific forms of instruction are only one form of experience, often inappropriate to practical action in immediate physical and social contexts unless one has been highly versed in such skills for years. Patients often founder with the task of thinking scientifically about their health problem because they do not have the appropriate skills, while scientific thinking has become the quasi-official definition of what they ought to learn.

The major focus of much instruction for patients might well be that of the craftsman—how to do, directed by thought.

SHARPNESS OF FOCUS OF INSTRUCTION

A number of instructional approaches are better able to produce a particular kind of learning than other kinds because they focus the learning activities on the behavior to be learned. Even such a broad approach as group discussion is usually directed at a particular kind of outcome, such as emotional support with some exchange of information, or at an opportunity to learn from one member of a group in order to model his behavior. Such a focused purpose is generally thought to be necessary in order to efficiently produce a specific behavior in a learner. In contrast, diffuseness means that all kinds of content and learning exercises are brought in without any clear notion of how they contribute to the behavior to be learned.

Nearly all useful behaviors consist of combinations of skills and attitudes. For example, carrying out a medication regimen can be broken into learning components and each brought into focus with supportive instruction (Table 6-3). It can be seen that each component also has subcomponents, some of which many patients may already have learned.

OVERCOMING LIMITATIONS OF A PARTICULAR LEARNING CONTEXT

Any episode of learning occurs in a specific situation and is profoundly influenced by that fact. Commonly, people have to use the skill in more situations

TABLE 6-3.
LEARNING COMPONENTS AND APPROPRIATE INSTRUCTIONAL ACTIVITY TO YIELD OUTCOME BEHAVIOR

End Outcome Behavior	Learning Component	Appropriate Instructional Activity
Carrying out medication regimen safely and accurately.	1. Understanding of how to take the medication and ability to recognize if its possible outcomes and side effects are occurring (if they can be sensed by the patient).	1. Written and oral giving of facts; practice in identifying effects.
	2. Desire to carry out the regimen which is seen in actually carrying it out.	2. Credible authority telling the patient to do regimen, or self-motivation boosted by feedback that he is doing the task right or it is making him feel better.
	3. Taking the medicine; for some medications there may be special skills of self-administration (injection) and measuring effect (taking own blood pressure).	3. Demonstration and practice and redemonstration of the skill, often accompanied by patient's explanation of actions.

than the one in which it was learned and may not be able to transfer the learning to the new situation.

There are several common approaches to dealing with this problem. Because they may be expensive, their use depends on how critical the needed skill is:

1. Provide multiple practice opportunities for the patient in multiple situations
2. Teach the skill in the context in which it will be used, not in a contrived context
3. Teach, also, people with whom the patient lives who may be better able to figure out how to make the transfer[6]

SUMMARY OF LEARNING AND TEACHING APPROACHES FOR PROCEDURES WITH MOTOR SKILLS

Most motor skills occur within procedures, which are a series of intellectually guided steps that yield a completed act. There are many such procedures in health; self-examination of the breast is an example. Component motor skills of a procedure have to be fully learned before the components can be put together. Motor skills improve with practice, often steadily over a long period of time if it is difficult for the learner to detect internal kinesthetic cues.

There are learning phases for such procedures, each providing different instructional support. The first phase is understanding the task. Teaching is often verbal or pictorial, directing a learner's attention to the proper sequence of action and to the cues that signal the start of each movement. Demonstrations provide a mental image of how to do the procedure and allow the learner to practice it mentally. In the second phase, partial skills are honed and put together in sequence. In the final phase, the learning becomes automatic, the learner does not have to think what to do next and he can be engaged in other activities at the same time. The skill increases in smoothness and precision. Practice and feedback about how to improve the skill are essential at this stage.[6]

Although direction on how to carry out elements of motor learning in patient education is clearly open to verification, such studies are not common. Such direction would especially be of use when the instruction is to be used at a future time in a different circumstance, and so observation of mastery is not possible. An example is the amount of practice of breathing and practice of neuromuscular release that would yield the best results for reducing pain in prepared childbirth. These exercises are part of the physiotherapy elements of childbirth education; other elements are didactic and attitudinal (fostering of a more positive attitude toward labor and birth). Studies done by Cogan[5] found that practice of neuromuscular release for 5 to 10 minutes a day and practice of breathing for 10 to 15 minutes a day by husbands and wives together seemed to provide an optimal foundation for childbirth preparation. Very limited practice time was associated with a real likelihood of increased pain during prepared birth.

SUMMARY OF LEARNING OF ATTITUDES

It appears that the conditions for learning attitudes are complex. Perhaps this is why most of our attitudes are learned incidentally rather than as a result of preplanned instruction. One of the most dependable events that has been found to produce changes in attitudes is human modeling. In these circumstances, learning results in imitation of an appealing and credible model's behavior.

SAMPLE METHODS USED IN PATIENT EDUCATION: ANALYSIS OF INSTRUCTIONAL ELEMENTS

Patient education has adopted some characteristic methods of instruction, although the frequency of their use is not known. Some are adaptations of methods used in schools or in public persuasion. Others reflect the delivery system of patient education including the necessity to negotiate a place for patient education. While not exhaustive, consideration of such methods allows analysis of their instructional characteristics.

VALUES CLARIFICATION

This is a method developed first for the school setting in response to concerns about affective education. It has been used in schools since 1970 and more recently is being adapted to patient settings.

Values clarification requires careful integration of knowledge, values, and decision making and uses loosely related techniques. These all require steps for understanding the issues, clarifying one's own values, making choices, knowing the consequences, and then making behavioral goals from those choices. For example, in the school setting, one exercise required students to evaluate 10 potential candidates for perpetuating the human race and to select 6 candidates. This required knowledge and value regarding fertility and genetics as a base. The role of the health educator is to use clarifying responses and the discussion of the strategy, such as, "What would be the consequences of that idea?" "What would you have to assume for things to work out that way?" In schools, this method has been used in the framework of the life-style curriculum, to assist in the evaluation and intelligent selection of the alternatives in life-style.[16]

This same method has also been used in an exploratory fashion with 20 chronic heart patients.[2] This use was based on the notion that heart disease necessitates adjustments in life-style that may come about more readily if patients are permitted to choose their own goals.

This program was based on steps of the valuing process (the steps one goes through in selecting personal values, including those about health) which involved choosing from alternatives after consideration of consequences, prizing and cherishing and publicly affirming, acting on one's choice finally, repetitively, and with consistency. A baseline assessment was done in areas of life-style change that often involve choice and conflicts for cardiac patients: smoking, work stress, physical activity, and diet. Four initial value-clarifying strategies were given to each patient, who then set a priority for changing his or her life-style. The patient was given four other value-clarifying strategies concerned primarily with the chosen priority area and then made an evaluation according to a set goal. The strategies in this study were in verbal and written form. One required a patient to list 20 cherished activities and place them within such categories as physical activities, those done in the prior two months, whether it cost money, those done with other people, and whether it involved eating. This strategy was to help patients examine their most prized and cherished activities that they still wanted to continue despite the limitations imposed by their heart condition.

The approach worked less well for patients who were heavily denying, those who were very ill, and those who chose not to change because of age.[2] Instructionally, values clarification includes providing facts, including probable consequences of particular events and actions. Its major thrust is providing a structure (the strategies) that make patients aware of their conflicts in the areas of life affected by the disease. It assists with motivated choices and goal setting and holds people accountable for their goals. It packages many of the areas necessary for informed behavior change.

MASS MEDIA APPROACHES

Telephone approaches and health fairs are selected for analysis. They clearly are not the most common mass media approaches but do represent different ways to further individualize instruction. For example, prepared telephone tapes allow the caller to focus on a topic of concern. In one such system that was oriented to cancer control, the most popular topics were smoking cessation and detection of cancer of the breast. Determination of content of the tapes can usually be assisted by an advisory committee.[21]

A more personal approach is the hotline concept, where instead of a taped message, the caller can get answers to direct questions. One such system operated by Monmouth Medical Center was designed to provide a link between untreated venereal disease patients and available medical services. The operators were trained in content and teaching approach. The most frequent in-quiries related to making clinic appointments and to the symptoms of the venereal disease.[3]

Health fairs can serve a variety of purposes such as making providers aware of community needs and consumers aware of community health resources, distributing health information including a directory of area health services, and offering some direct services such as immunizations and diagnostic test-ing. A definition of health will also serve in deciding about agencies and dis-plays to accept.[19]

Besides the opportunity to individualize more than the true mass media approach, hotlines and health fairs can provide somewhat anonymous access to persons and information.

WRITTEN MATERIALS

A great deal of health and patient education utilizes pamphlets, health product inserts, and so forth. The client may choose materials himself, or they may be prescribed for him. For example, the popular literature on child care alone is immense: it is estimated that the number of child care books sold in the United States in the past 5 years is about 23 million. A limited survey of Chicago residents who read such books found that the books gave them a better under-standing of child development but were less effective in changing the child's behavior.[4] The books were criticized for being too permissive, not practical or specific enough especially for individual differences in child development or familial circumstances. It might be surmised that people turn to such books to substitute for information from personal networks. Based on this limited sur-vey, there is clearly room for improvement in the quality of the literature on child care.[4]

A major limitation with use of such materials is that some clients are poor readers and/or are not motivated to learn from such materials. As with mass media approaches, there is not a large prescriptive literature (research-tested methods) for design of effective materials. There are, however, well known methods of product (educational) evaluation that lead to improvement and retesting until one is satisfied with or abandons the product.

Probably because of the relatively unsystematic approach (from an educa-tional view) to the overall development of materials for a field, it is not un-common to find a dearth of such materials for a subpopulation and/or subject matter. An example is educational materials for pregnant teenagers, includ-ing such subjects as the early symptoms of pregnancy, how to get a pregnancy test, the possibility of miscarriage, and how to get job, child care, and educa-tional counseling as well as medical care and economic help.[1]

Drug labeling and patient package inserts are tools for patient education; their effectiveness needs also to be tested.

DEMONSTRATION AND PARTICIPATION IN CARE

This can be a relatively formal or informal method of great importance since patients many times have to be trained to carry out procedures on their own. For example, the mirror pelvic exam is a kind of patient-participatory education aimed at increasing women's knowledge of their anatomy and making the procedure less anxiety provoking. The mirror pelvic exam consists of a routine pelvic examination modified only by having the patient elevate her head and shoulders by propping herself up on one elbow. With the other hand she holds a mirror between her legs to one side of the midline, positioned to visualize first her external genitalia and, following speculum insertion her vaginal walls and cervix. Dialogue between the patient and examiner accompanies this procedure so that anatomic characteristics can be identified and described, allowing opportunity for questions and answers. One clinical survey found this opportunity to be viewed positively by patients, contributing to relaxation and reduced fears,[12] although the degree to which this finding can be generalized is not known.

Patients and family members have been trained to do a variety of medical procedures for themselves that vary in the degree of risk and skill. One such example is the resuscitation of infants with life-threatening apnea caused by near-miss sudden infant death syndrome at home. The parents were instructed in use of an apnea monitor and in resuscitation. Although the survival rate was 93 percent, some infants had repeated instances of apnea. Experience of this group indicated that supervision of this home monitoring should include 24-hour availability of medical, technical, and counseling assistance.[10] In this instance, the home monitoring became the real learning experience, with initial learning of the procedures far less stressful than carrying them out with one's own infant at home. Such demonstration and participation have the strength of realism and motivation. These are often very potent learning experiences and so can have potent side effects, such as tremendous anxiety that causes the procedure to be performed incorrectly. These need to be monitored carefully.

PROGRAMS

Many times instruction is organized within a health or community institution to give it coherence and visibility. This is especially true when patients need to learn complex skills. Besides coherence in learning, there are often political reasons for such organization. Such a structure allows negotiation for the introduction and maintenance of a program that may have been foreign to such a setting and that has a high probability of being resisted by some member.

An example of a special program developed as a field demonstration is the parent–child development center program. First started in three cities in the United States, the goal was parent education for low-income mothers and children up to three years old. Also available were other supportive social and medical services such as instruction in homemaking, driver education, and courses for high school credit aimed at supporting parents by helping people gain control over their own lives. A laboratory setting for practicing parenting skills and gaining feedback through videotapes provided an important instructional means.[8]

In health settings, patient education programs are common, although not comprehensive. In community hospitals, concerns regarding length of stay and liability regarding informed consent have been an impetus to patient education, although physician referral of individual patients is still a common method for participation. One hospital offers group classes for patients with diabetes, emphysema, hypertension, heart disease, preoperative and renal dialysis, patient clubs, volunteer visits, individual instruction, community health education aimed primarily at prevention, screening and detection programs, and use of video and written materials. Such programs are often experimenting with a variety of approaches.[11]

Description is also available regarding the process of setting up programs, for example, for diabetes instruction in hospitals and learning centers in clinics.[9] Diabetes classes covering different topics each day and repeated weekly for in- and outpatients are common. Visiting nurse referral for follow-up helps complete the learning. While nurses often do much of the teaching in such programs and coordinate it, decisions regarding the program are commonly made by many disciplines but especially by medicine.[15] Organization into programs tells nothing about the basic mechanisms for instruction.

CURRICULA OF PATIENT EDUCATION PROGRAMS

Any instruction that is more than brief takes on the characteristics of a curriculum and uses structuring and selection criteria for the content. These decisions are often determined by negotiation among a group of health specialists. Curriculum is primarily concerned with content while instruction is concerned with teaching approach, and they can to some extent be separated.

A survey intended to identify the nature and extent of consumer health education programming in the United States with a particular focus on evaluation found that few health education programs exist for a long period of time. Very few programs had been in operation continuously for more than two years; the large majority seemed to be short-term programs that operated at most over a period of three to four months and usually over an even shorter period.[13] This is too short a time to produce systematic concern by a stable group of people concerning the makeup of the curriculum. When conceptualized and described, the curriculum can often be improved.

In the specialized books of this series, reference will be made to decisions about selection of content and conceptual structure in which it will be presented and to sequencing of content. Curricula can be described by content inclusion and emphasis. They can also be described longitudinally as a naturalistic case study. Identification of difficulties and development of solutions tend to be worked out over a period of time in a series of partial reformulations. There is a steady refashioning and unfolding of the ideas with an internal logic, and there are stages of deliberation and negotiation. The patient education literature is nearly devoid of such descriptive case studies, which could serve to make the innovative solutions and processes available to others and serve as a descriptive research base. Some conceptual framework is implicit in any program of instruction; it can be elucidated by examination of the selection and structuring criteria with such questions as: Is it oriented to the physician's regimen, at least in part because physicians are commonly the persons who determine content to be taught? Is the framework management of daily living, with items of the regimen incorporated into this larger structure?[18] Are there concepts simple enough for many to understand, or are there ways to simplify the requirements for time, commitment, and technical knowledge?

The concerns of curriculum, then, are complementary to those of instruction and require analysis and management. A program is not only formal and used with a group but also can be sequential teaching with individual patients as they come on the service, using a common protocol. Of considerable concern, also, is the freedom for the nurse to function at a professional level in joint decision-making about curricular elements.

SUMMARY

Instruction involves making judgments on the kind of directed learning that fits both the task to be learned and the patient's abilities. While certain general approaches and methods have developed, differentiation among them is made by analysis of the activities they direct the learner to do.

REFERENCES

1. Ambrose, L. Mis-informing pregnant teenagers. *Family Planning Perspectives*, 1978, *10*, 51–57.
2. Berger, B., Hopp, J. W., & Raettig, V. Values clarification in the cardiac patient. *Health Education Monographs*, 1975, *3*, 191–199.
3. Bryant, N. H., Stender, W., Frist, W., & Somers, A. VD hotline: an evaluation. *Public Health Reports*, 1976, *91*, 231–235.
4. Clarke-Steward, K. A. Popular primers for parents. *American Psychologist*, 1978, *33*, 359–369.
5. Cogan, R. Practice time in prepared childbirth. *Journal of Obstetric and Gynecologic Nursing*, 1978, *7(1)*, 33–38.
6. Gagne, R. M. *The conditions of learning*, 3rd ed. New York: Holt, 1977.
7. Goldstein, M. K., Stein, G. H., Smolen, D. M., & Perlini, W. S. Bio-behavioral monitoring: a method for remote health mesurement. *Archives of Physical Medicine and Rehabilitation*, 1976, *57*, 253–258.

8. Gross, B., & Gross, R. Parent-child development center: creating models for parent education. *Children Today,* 1977, *6,* 18–22.

9. Hoffman, L. E., Jr. Patient education: how we designed our own program. *Group Practice,* 1976, *25(5),* 21–24.

10. Kelly, D. H., Shannon, D. C., & O'Connell, K. Care of infants with near-miss sudden infant death syndrome. *Pediatrics,* 1978, *61,* 511–514.

11. Lane, D. S. Patient education in the community hospital. *Journal of Biocommunication,* 1978, *5,* 6–10.

12. Liston, J., & Liston, E. H., Jr. The mirror pelvic examination: assessment in a clinical setting. *Journal of Obstetric and Gynecologic Nursing,* 1978, *7(2),* 47–49.

13. Little AD Inc: *Executive summary: A survey of consumer health education programs.* DHEW Contract 100-75-0082, 1976.

14. Lundberg, M. J. *The incomplete adult; social class constraints on personality development.* Westport, Conn.: Greenwood Press, 1974.

15. Manfredi, C., Cassity, V., & Moffitt, B. D. Developing a teaching program for diabetic mothers. *Journal of Continuing Education in Nursing,* 1977, *8(6),* 46–52.

16. Meeks, L. The use and abuse of values clarification in the life style approach to health education. *Health Values: Achieving High Level Wellness,* 1977, *1,* 82–85.

17. Olson, D. R. The language of instruction: the literate bias of schooling. In Anderson, R. C., & Spiro, R. J. (Eds.). *Schooling and the acquisition of knowledge.* Hillsdale, N. J.: Lawrence Erlbaum, 1977.

18. Redman, B. K. On the concept of curriculum in patient education. *American Journal of Nursing,* 1978, *78,* 1363–1365.

19. Richie, N. D. Some guidelines for conducting a health fair. *Public Health Reports,* 1976, *91,* 261–274.

20. Shuell, T. J., & Lee, C. Z. *Learning and instruction.* Monterey, Cal.: Brooks/Cole, 1976.

21. Wilkinson, G. S., Mirand, E. A., & Graham, S. Can-dial: An experiment in health education and cancer control. *Public Health Reports,* 1976, *91,* 218–222.

7
DIFFERENTIATING TEACHING AND OTHER PSYCHOSOCIAL INTERVENTIONS

There is a wide range of psychosocial intervention strategies available, with varying degrees of overlap in purpose and methods. Generally, their separation has occurred by their theoretical bases. In the health field, psychiatry has formed the umbrella for most behavioral issues, especially for individuals, and public health focuses on health of populations, using the epidemiologic model and public health education as one intervention strategy.

Definition of education of individuals in clinical situations has not been clear, and this area of practice has not had a home. The tendency was for it to be subsumed under the predominant field of thought: psychiatric theory in psychiatry and the public health perspective in public health. Neither did it justice and seem to put forward an incomplete or out-of-date perspective on teaching. As an example, a 1977 textbook on psychotherapy indicates that even though education has focused on the development of the intellectual capacities of the individual and his acquisition of knowledge, a new direction in the purpose of education has been extended to include emotional growth of the individual.[9] Emotional growth, however, has been part of educational theory for centuries.

COMPARISON OF CLASSES OF PSYCHOSOCIAL INTERVENTION APPROACHES

Table 7-1 describes in gross form the author's conception of differentiation between teaching, psychotherapy, and behavioral intervention approaches.

Emotional problems can block learning so teaching has tried to deal with such blocks. When they become severe, however, teaching is not seen as the primary therapy, and they often disrupt the learning process in a school.

The field of education has well-developed strategies for accumulating knowledge, developing intellectual and physical skills, and assisting with moral and emotional development. These are most highly developed within the

TABLE 7-1.
ROUGH COMPARISON OF CLASSES OF PSYCHOSOCIAL INTERVENTION
APPROACHES

	Teaching	Psychotherapy	Behavioral Approaches
Populations	Normal	Those distorting reality* as in crisis or longer term, and socially disruptive persons	All of these
Primary therapeutic thrust	Development of understanding and cognitive/psychomotor skills	Emotions including those affected by others, taking into account cognition	Behavior change, using internal and external environment as reinforcers. In the process, thoughts and emotions change.
Estimated motivational power in health situations	Adequate when problem responds to this therapeutic thrust. Usually necessary but not sufficient in major behavior changes. A major source of motivation seen to be feelings of competence from mastering ideas and skills, and to a lesser extent relationship with teacher.	Strength or power not clear. Major source of motivation seen to be relationship with therapist.	Motivation defined as reinforcement. Ability to sustain this reinforcement variable.
Incorporation into nursing process	Could be nearly complete except for patients with special learning and readiness problems. Teaching can be served appropriately by a nurse specially prepared at Master's level. Physicians still generally determine content to be taught.	Generally seen as appropriate for Master's-prepared specialist. General supportive process seen as appropriate for RN.	Irregularly incorporated into specialty practice in nursing, as in the field of mental retardation. Basic principles should be integrated and used at all levels of nursing. The independent role is still seen as largely that of the psychologic worker.

*Promoting mental health, also seen as an important goal of psychiatric/mental health workers, deals with normal persons and uses methods more akin to those of teaching, plus additional environmental support.

Note: All three of these classes are not primarily dependent on physiologic learning as is, for example, biofeedback.

purposes, environment, and subject group of the school. Within the health field, experience has exposed some of the limits of education. For example, life-style changes probably cannot be brought about through the traditional approaches of education alone. Likewise, some orientations to psychotherapy see skill development as critical, both to care of the emotionally disturbed person and in preventive mental health to allow the patient to be more productive and capable. Persons concerned with psychological rehabilitation believe that training should be used to provide the disabled persons with the physical, intellectual, and emotional skills needed to live in the community with the least possible support from agents from the helping professions. This is more analogous to the rehabilitation approach used in physical medicine rather than similar to many current psychiatric treatment approaches such as psychoanalysis and other insight-oriented therapies.[1]

Although education has focused heavily on cognition, cognitive explanations of psychiatric disorders is not uncommon. Cognition is thought to determine affect and is a broad term that refers to both the content of thought and the processes involved in thinking. Ways of perceiving and processing material, the mechanisms and content of memory and recall, and problem-solving attitudes are all aspects of cognition. Cognitive structures are relatively enduring characteristics of a person's cognitive organization, and the schemas used in them may be complex, multifaceted, and well-developed or not.

The cognitive approach to psychiatric illness tries to alter or remove only those thought patterns that are pathogenic, such as the negative value judgments of depression, which often remain relatively immune to conventional corrective feedback (although there may well have been lack of opportunity to submit them to examination). The individual is preoccupied with self-derogatory and self-blaming thoughts, selectively recalls such material, and draws conclusions in the absence of or contrary to evidence. Intervention includes planning productive activities to break the depressive circle and providing the patient with experiences of accomplishment and pinpointing the distorted cognitions and modifying the thinking errors.[4]

So instruction is not seen as a "deep" therapeutic agent with psychiatric patients. It is not primarily aimed at psychological insight. Explanation and clarification can function as effective curative agents in relieving anxiety from uncertainty and can be used with psychiatric patients, especially in those areas of their lives that are not disturbed.

Regarding theoretical base, the use of psychoanalytic theories has not been predominant in education, which has used instead general learning theories, seen to best fit the tasks and subjects of school learning. Behavioral approaches have come from social learning theory, especially in the form of operant conditioning and have been applied in both psychiatry and education. Such skills are, however, less well integrated at any level of depth into education, and this model is not commonly the only theory used in educational settings.

Biofeedback and relaxation training are also considered to be behavioral methods although with a firmer physiologic base. These approaches, including operant conditioning, have been applied to headaches, type A behavior patterns, insomnia, obesity, urinary disorders, cardiac arrhythmias, hypertension, and others.[8] Some of the better established of these techniques can be incorporated into the general practice of nursing.

Primary prevention and health promotion in mental health converge closely with an educational model, which perhaps explains their less than complete integration into psychiatry. They are aimed at improving levels of functioning and at dealing with obstacles to that functioning. In primary prevention, the strategies are directed toward persons in stress or at risk in one or more of the domains of living. The strategies are directed toward helping the individual at risk to either avoid the risk or better cope with it. These may be educational strategies (sometimes called anticipatory guidance), developmental strategies, consultation, and supportive intervention at the time of crisis. Strategies directed toward the environment reduce rules and restrictions, increase resources so people can better meet their needs, and remove noxious agents such as noise that put people at risk. Simply improving the quality of life for individuals is seen to be an effective strategy for primary prevention.[5]

In promotion of positive mental health, the goal is comparable to programs of physical fitness and nutrition which are targeted to improve performance rather than those special programs directed at preventing specific clinical disorders. The strategies are directed at persons in situations of normal growth and development to improve their functioning. The strategies are again educational, developmental, and environmental.[5]

With the exception of the social welfare components, these programs share both goals and intervention strategies with teaching. What does it matter if the program is given to improve mental health or to improve competence in a role (education)? Improved mental health is often an outcome of an educational program that provides competencies and confidence.

In summary, education in health areas has rarely been a direct intervention method to alter a disease process. It is almost always necessary for assisting with adjustment to or development of behaviors necessary to a physical or chemical treatment regimen, or in producing preventive behaviors. These can vary from understanding the treatment, to having the skills and judgment to carry it out on one's self or on a family member. Education can be a direct intervention for producing preventive health behaviors.

A final word should be said about casting educational interventions in their most narrow form, sometimes as a way of isolating approaches in research projects. In a particular study aimed at assisting patients to comply with their hypertensive regimens, social support groups were compared with a program of lecture sessions. In explaining the conclusion that no differences could be found between these groups but that both were superior to the control or "standard treatment group," the author cites data that perhaps the lecture group had been run in a little too supportive a manner to introduce clear differences between it and the social support group.[2] This is not unexpected; given the nature of the behavior to be obtained, no self-respecting patient education program would have used a purely factual approach.

From a medical point of view, patient education has mostly been supportive therapy, although from a holistic point of view it has been a critical element of other therapies. Consider the conception by Nancy Keller,[3] which starts with the position that consumers often receive little or no information which helps them feel in command of themselves in certain situations. She suggests the usefulness of an information broker, working consistently at providing options and accurate information and at verifying or correcting the client's impressions. The client is given information and assistance, he processes it into options acceptable within his life-style and anticipatory of daily events, integrates it with his structure of meaning, and is ready to act as his own advocate for obtaining what help he needs.

AN ECLECTIC MODEL FOR PSYCHOSOCIAL NURSING

There are groups of patients who require a purely psychiatric model (e.g., those emotionally disturbed) and those for whom a purely teaching model has been successful (e.g., normal prenatal instruction). Many kinds of patient situations, especially over time for particular patients, require less pure models since health matters, including illness, are emotional for many and disrupt usual living patterns. Psychosocial care for most requires combination interventions that provide cognitive, affective, and behavioral approaches. At points in time, the patient may require both educational and psychiatric approaches perhaps given by different persons.

Training for home dialysis requires a large affective component in what is conceived to be primarily a teaching (knowledge and skill) development approach. This is an emotionally laden situation, and at times the patient may become disturbed enough to require psychiatric intervention. In genetic counseling, clinical acuity in assessing the possibility of emotional hazards is essential, and psychiatric training is useful.

One study of patients who used excessive denial as a defense in the acute phase of coronary care found that such patients have considerable subsequent vulnerability to disruptive anxiety and depression. Management of such patients included first brief psychotherapy to support self-esteem while confronting fear of death, uncertainty of recurrence, and threat of lost function. Then cardiac rehabilitation (education and mobilization) was used to prevent reassertion of the denial by requiring action and showing measured physical progress.[7]

An additional example is that of counseling rape victims and their families. Although seen primarily as counseling within a crisis framework, educating the people close to the victim about the nature of the crisis she is experiencing and helping them to anticipate future likely psychological and somatic sequelae is as much a part of treatment as is encouraging family members to express their own affective responses to the trauma and providing counseling to those whose responses are so profound as to affect their own ability to cope adequately.[6]

The changes in behavior that patients need to accomplish can be seen as the combination of cognitive, affective, and skill learning. Each is present to some degree and to some level of complexity. The emphasis placed on any particular element depends primarily on the orientation of the professional in charge since each may operate under theories that conceptualize behavioral tasks differently and the way to deal with them. For example, many psychiatric theories intend to make changes in the patient's thinking but approach it through the affective realm, which is seen to be primary.

Educational approaches have been strongest for cognitive learning and for some skill learning, primarily motor. Psychological or psychiatric thought has been strongest in the affective and social skills realms. It is useful for nonpsychiatric patients, i.e., those basically competent and in touch with reality, to consciously choose from the wide variety of psychosocial approaches. Thus, one may not see oneself as doing patient teaching unless the patient problem and one's orientation can draw primarily from the teaching approach. When counseling or "doing therapy," one may also be using elements of patient teaching.

We do not have a good descriptive verb for this kind of combination therapy; it is commonly called providing psychosocial care. There are those who believe that a good quality helping relationship is the basis of psychosocial care and that it does not matter much by which theoretical approach the helping relationship is enacted. Others believe that particular approaches are focused and therefore are better able to create certain kinds of behavior change than do other approaches.

At any rate, this author believes the approaches to be complementary, sometimes overlapping, but clearly in need of conceptual separation and analysis to clarify the field.

REFERENCES

1. Anthony, W. A. Psychological rehabilitation: A concept in need of a method. *American Psychologist,* 1977, *32,* 658–662.
2. Caplan, R. D., Robinson, E. A. R., French, J. R. P., Caldwell, J. R., & Shinn, M. *Adhering to medical regimens: Pilot experiments in patient education and social support.* Ann Arbor: Institute for Social Research, University of Michigan, 1976.
3. Keller, N. S. Private nursing practice: some facilitators and barriers in health care. In Leininger, M. (Ed.). *Barriers and facilitators to quality health care.* Philadelphia: Davis, 1975.
4. Kovacs, M., & Beck, A. T. Maladaptive cognitive structures in depression. *American Journal of Psychiatry,* 1978, *135,* 525–533.
5. McPheeters, H. L. Primary prevention and health promotion in mental health. *Preventive Medicine,* 1976, *5,* 187–198.
6. Silverman, D. C. Sharing the crisis of rape: Counseling the mates and families of victims. *American Journal of Orthopsychiatry,* 1978, *48,* 166–173.
7. Soloff, P. H. Denial and rehabilitation of the postinfarction patient. *International Journal of Psychiatry in Medicine,* 1978, *8,* 125–132.
8. Williams, R. B., Jr., & Gentry, W. D. *Behavioral approaches to medical treatment.* Cambridge, Ma.: Ballinger, 1977.
9. Wolberg, I. R. *The technique of psychotherapy, part I,* 3rd ed. New York: Grune & Stratton, 1977.

8

POTENTIAL NEGATIVE SIDE EFFECTS

Patient education is now explicitly included in many Nurse Practice Acts. In this author's opinion, it is in the process of evolving into a truly therapeutic tool, practiced at a professional level.

One of the barriers to that evolvement is some confused thinking when determining the occurrence and frequency of negative side effects. This occurs for at least two reasons:

1. There is a notion that education is either beneficial for a patient or has no effect at all. Although this is not true, clarity about what those negative side effects can be is not common.
2. Evaluation is, perhaps, the part of the patient teaching process that is performed most poorly. There are few tools for evaluation, most of whose reliability and validity have not been studied. Evaluation appears not to be commonly done and very rarely for the full time span that a particular teaching intervention has its effect. But perhaps more important is the fact that the purpose of most evaluation in this field is still seen as determining the degree to which *intended* effects (those laid out as objectives) have occurred. It is rare that unintended effects are monitored; yet they can be more beneficial or more devastating than are intended effects.

It is, therefore, unclear how frequently negative side effects occur; yet monitoring for them and taking corrective action when they occur is essential to making patient teaching a safer, more highly therapeutic treatment.

KINDS OF NEGATIVE SIDE EFFECTS

The judgment that an effect is negative or undesirable is, of course, relative. But the following would be considered negative by professional judgment:

1. Incorrect information or skills on which the patient acts. This includes wrong specific information such as how much medication to take. It also includes creation of incorrect perspectives or expectations (combination of information or attitude), e.g., about the range of treatment options or the likelihood of complications occurring in a person with a chronic disease. This forms a set that may well influence the patient's life goals. The source of such errors is often difficult to trace since a certain amount of distortion of reality is common in persons under crisis, those dealing with information overload and sometimes with a physiologic basis for decreased memory, problem-solving capacity, and so on.

2. Creation of undesirable attitudinal motivational state.   Confusion, lack of confidence, and anxiety can be incapacitating. These states can be created by an educational intervention that creates information overload that cannot be processed and by the communicated feeling that the patient is not competent, especially in a patient who is functioning minimally. In addition, anxiety can be excessive if the teaching threatens the mechanism by which a patient has been coping with psychological problems. And a patient can vow to avoid any future education after a traumatic learning experience.

Some fear that overdependence can be produced by patient education. The obvious way to avoid that is to create an implicit or an explicit contract with the patient that requires him to take increasing responsibility for his own behavior. Guilt can be created when the patient knows he is deviating from professional norms, which could lead to preoccupation with illness and inferiority. There is some evidence that knowledge about drugs such as alcohol and amphetamines, marijuana, barbiturates, and LSD is significantly related to use.[1] Whether the knowledge causes the use is not yet clear.

3. Imposition of behavioral norms for one cultural group on persons from another.   This side effect affects both individuals and entire groups. There have been questions about whether some patterns of health behavior expected by health professionals were really not empirically based and reflected middle-class norms.[2] These can be imposed on other groups through teaching and attempting to create those expected behaviors.

4. Delay of constructive social action.   Health education can be used as a way to avoid dealing with hard questions of social justice and social policy. "Educating the public" about a matter such as alcohol abuse with unreal expectations of outcome is an example of such avoidance.[3]

MONITORING PLANS

Some of these negative side effects can be monitored concurrently with delivery of the teaching intervention. Getting feedback from the patient about how well he can perform the tasks he is trying to learn is essential for redirecting the teaching intervention. This practice also allows the nurse to identify incorrect perceptions, information, and skills the patient is learning. So, also, can some of the undesirable mental states be immediately identified. Some, however, occur when the patient moves from a protected environment such as the hospital into his usual living pattern, or when he encounters stress in his life and increased coping abilities are required.

Longer-term monitoring plans are difficult because patient education is rarely conceived as an intermittently delivered but planned and accumulative intervention. It is often so diffuse that linking it with a particular patient outcome is difficult. This has particular salience for teaching since patients learn about health matters from sources other than the professional. Just as they take drugs on their own advice or that of others, so do they learn. But a first step is an ongoing monitoring of those for whom patient education is a major and/or ongoing therapeutic intervention. Most persons with chronic illness are in this category. This allows identification and correction of these side effects as well as those from other treatments the patient is receiving.

A different level of monitoring is required for patient education which is accomplished by means often remote to large numbers of people. The preparation of educational literature for mass distribution is an example of this approach. Educational product development techniques are well known in the field of education but almost never used for health materials. Although still inexact, such techniques require testing the intended and unintended effects of educational materials on pilot groups of persons for whom the material is meant, with constant refinement until tests show positive outcomes.

Such materials (pamphlets) should be tested as self-instructional, by the educational impact they create by themselves, although at times they may be used with other methods of instruction such as a teacher. Critiques of entire bodies of literature, such as the audiovisual and printed materials largely produced by industry, that educate adolescents on menstruation for instance, are available. Probably because they are meant to sell products, such materials have approached the subject of menarche principally from the viewpoint of hygiene. One critique found them to convey the view that menstruation is similar to a sickness and akin to excretory soiling; the materials were also found to focus on reproduction as the essence of the change at menarche, and to focus on hygiene rules.[5,6] These publications are limited in their focus on menarche, because information on female physiology and the emotional changes which occur as a result of menarche were not presented.

TEACHING AS A VEHICLE FOR A PARTICULAR MEDICAL TREATMENT PLAN

Negative side effects from the process of teaching are not to be confused with the side effects from the medical regimen which patients have been taught to carry out. It is clear, however, that difficulties with self-administration of the medical regimen do create anxieties and lack of confidence that affect the ability and interest in learning. This situation is not uncommon.

For the ten leading causes of death from disease in the United States, "halfway" technologies, representing the best available treatment but not capable of turning off, reversing, or preventing disease, are most of what is available. For example, cancer treatments such as surgery, radiation, chemotherapy, and immunotherapy cannot reverse or prevent the neoplastic process but rather try to control it by destroying cells.[4] In addition, these "halfway" technologies (ability to control but not cure) vary in their effectiveness in controlling disease and in the side effects they produce. Some require long-term self-administration of a medical treatment regimen, such as the diabetes regimen and home hemodialysis for kidney disease. It ought to be noted that predictions of our ability to get people to learn to self-administer a particular technology are not commonly part of the decision to adopt it on a broad scale. Neither is there much control of the educative function to see that the teaching methods developed are effective for persons from the broad range of socioeconomic status. This failure makes for inequitable access to the technologies.

Because halfway technologies, which form the content of some teaching, are so common, a certain range of side effects will commonly be seen in teaching programs, related largely to the prognosis and to the onerousness of the self-care involved. Examples are anxiety about the course of the disease and the degree to which the regimen is controlling it and depression related to the alteration in life-style created by the social and physical effects of the regimen.

Some also believe that in recent years the public's perception of its own health has changed as seen from this quote:

Left alone, unadvised by a professional, the tendency of the human body is perceived as prone to steady failure . . . it needs to be said more often that human beings are fundamentally tough.[4]

This situation, if true, can lead to "overteach," an expansion of patient education so that large numbers of people can be taught to seek and carry out the services that are in question. While it is unlikely that halfway technology should or would be given up until something better is available, it is suggested by many that we should eliminate areas of health care in which spending of money represents outright waste.[3] This would also eliminate the teaching related to these areas; "overteach" can obviously be a negative side effect.

SUMMARY

Teaching, at this point in its evolution, is an inexact science. For this reason, effects cannot be predicted with a high degree of reliability. Possible negative side effects include patient action on incorrect information given by the professional; creation of undesirable mental states such as incapacitating confusion, killing of motivation and/or confidence; or creating the knowledge and a set to take undesirable action such as drug abuse. Monitoring with the set to tap unintended as well as intended effects of teaching can be done. Some negative effects occur because many of the medical technologies available are "half-way technologies," not entirely effective in controlling the disease and creating negative physical and social side effects.

REFERENCES

1. Halpin, G., and Whiddon, T. Drug education: Solution or problem? *Psychological Reports,* 1977, *40,* 372–374.
2. Milio, N. Values, social class and community health services. *Nursing Research,* 1967, *16,* 26–30.
3. Simonds, S. K. Health, values and ethics—an editorial opinion. *Health Values: Achieving High Level Wellness,* 1977, *1,* 99.
4. Thomas, L. On the science and technology of medicine. In Knowles, J. H. (Ed.). *Doing better and feeling worse.* New York: Norton, 1977.
5. Whisnant, L., & Zegans, L. Study of attitudes toward menarche in white middle-class American adolescent girls. *American Journal of Psychiatry,* 1975, *132,* 809–814.
6. Whisnant, L., Brett, E., & Zegans, L. Implicit messages concerning menstruation in commercial educational materials prepared for young adolescent girls. *American Journal of Psychiatry,* 1975, *132,* 815–820.

9
CRITERIA FOR QUALITY PATIENT EDUCATION

With pressures building to make patient education services more available, criteria of quality in that service becomes crucial. It seems to this author that clarity in this area is still developing and that lack of confidence in the health professions' ability to provide a high-quality service is a consequence.

A very simple structure for conceptualizing criteria for quality of patient education occurs in Table 9-1. Consideration of process and outcome is a key area of concern for patient education, since outcome standards are not well established in a number of behavior areas where teaching is being applied. The unit of delivery is singled out as the second dimension to be addressed because it is basic in conceptualizing a whole system of care, and each unit suffers from particular difficulties and requirements.

UNITS OF DELIVERY IN PATIENT EDUCATION

Because of its pervasiveness in patient care and the nature of the barriers to its proper performance, patient education needs to be viewed from several levels of service delivery.

Individual Patient. Deliberate patient education is used when a care-giver consciously attempts to alter a patient's behavior through the use of techniques more commonly identified with teaching than with other interpersonal therapies.

Programs of Patient Education. A program exists when one teaching protocol (including content) is applied to a number of patients. The clearest example of a program occurs when all the clients gather together in one place to receive the instruction. Since one often needs to identify how well a common protocol is working, however, it is useful to think of the summation of all instances of use of the protocol as also constituting a program, even though the care may be delivered to one patient at a time. Programs are especially vulnerable when there is confusion about criteria of quality of care. This occurs because they are identifiable entities with personnel assigned to them and often with a separate budget supporting the enterprise.

TABLE 9-1.
STRUCTURE FOR EVALUATION OF PATIENT
EDUCATION

Unit of Delivery	Kinds of Standards	
	Process	*Outcome*
Individual patient	Cell 1	Cell 2
Program of patient education	Cell 3	Cell 4
System for patient education	Cell 5	Cell 6

A System for Delivery of Patient Education. This level of structure seems necessary to consider since it is the place where decisions are made about what
patient education services are to be offered. These decisions, plus the overall
posture of the system regarding patient participation and access to advice
and teaching from professionals, create or remove barriers to patient education. Indeed, lack of patient access to health information can be a major block
to meeting proper outcome goals.

KINDS OF STANDARDS

Process standards simply describe how the activity ought to be carried out by
the health care-giver. An example would be a written teaching plan utilizing
information on the patient's readiness to learn.

Outcome standards describe the degree to which it is expected that the
desired goals for the patient can be reached. Green[5] describes six general
standards of acceptability for patient education outcomes, which he found
used, often implicitly, in studies in the literature.

1. *Historical standards.* Comparison at different points in time for the individual, the population, the problem, the program, or the technique.
2. *Normative standards.* Comparison with outcomes from another program,
   which are often in the same region. The ideal comparison group is the true
   control group in an experimental design.
3. *Absolute standards.* Set by policy decision makers as, perhaps, a 100 percent solution even though that may be unrealistic.
4. *Theoretical standards.* Based on what theory would predict should happen
   and on previous research.
5. *Negotiated standards.* Usually somewhere between the theoretical standard and the absolute standard, the compromise made through negotiation.
6. *Arbitrary standards.* Usually based on no information.

Green's work focused on the origins of standards. An example may be physicians' perceptions of present standards of informed consent, sometimes covered

by state law. These new standards may be viewed as absolute or arbitrary, while practitioners feel they should be normative, to take into account the fact that patients often do not listen to explanations, do not remember them, or perceive that what they recall is incorrect. A study of such problems with patients who had undergone open heart surgery found that accurate recall of less than 50 percent of the material was not uncommon, with some persons denying that topics had been discussed at all.[7] Obviously, the process the physician used needs to be examined to obtain better results, but so also does the probability that one could get total recall of information basic to informed consent.

Studies of the ability of lay people to perform care usually done by professionals commonly use normative standards. For example, one study showed parents at home able to detect streptococcal infections equally as frequently as health assistants in the clinic by obtaining throat cultures from their children.[9] Ability to teach this level of competence at least to certain groups of lay persons is not uncommon. Other criteria such as cost and satisfaction then also become important to consider.

Access to information about success rate is sometimes difficult to obtain. Many people are not keen to let others know about their failures, and the rates are often not commonly defined and cannot be compared. However, normative standards based on clinical experience at various sites are common. An example is the experience of a group teaching patients in the ghetto how to perform home dialysis. Their judgment is that more than 50 percent of such patients can be successfully trained and maintained.[1]

SUGGESTED SAMPLE PROCESS STANDARDS

Perhaps the use of process standards is more important than one would think because of the evidence that many patient education programs are not potent enough to cause the desired behavior change.[5,6] Lack of adequate potency can occur, for example, when there is insufficient practice to master the behavior, the instruction is not matched to the patient's readiness to learn, attention is not paid to how the behavior will be maintained over time, attitudes are not addressed although crucial to the behavior, social supports are not provided to aid retention of the behavior, the relationship with the health care-giver is formal, distant, and not open so a relationship of rapport does not develop (Fig. 9-1).

For individual patients (Cell 1 in Table 9-1), using elements of the teaching-
   learning process:
   Readiness (motivation and already existing knowledge, skills, and attitudes)
      Use natural readiness when available
         If necessary, stimulate readiness
      Setting objectives
      Match readiness with the outcome desired for health

**Increasing
amounts of time**

Temporary and noncritical information use

Written or oral instruction

·
·
·
·
·
·
·

·
·
·
·
·
·
·

Multiple basic behavior changes

Multiple teaching methods including relationship with teacher, involvement with
family and social environment

Figure 9-1.
Instructional potency continuum.

Providing instruction
  Use appropriately potent methods (see Fig. 9-1)
  Use techniques necessary for the kind of learning. *Example:* For motor
    skills, provide a mental image of the skill, reinforce practice with feed-
    back and correction
Evaluation of learning
  Have the patient perform the behavior, but if this is not possible, use the
    best simulated situation
  If the behavior is crucial, observe it many times in situations like those in
    which it will be used
  Test for both expected and unexpected effects
For programs (Cell 3 in Table 9-1), one needs to determine the degree to which
  the process standards for individual patients were carried out for all of the
  multiple patients in the program.
For delivery systems (Cell 5 in Table 9-1), there should be demonstration of
  monitoring and removal of barriers to proper patient access to health information; there should be a plan for delivery of patient education in that
  system, with evidence that there are competent people to carry it out

OUTCOME STANDARDS

Outcome standards will be considered in all of the books in this series, specific
to patients with particular learning goals required by treatment or prevention
of certain disease processes and health problems.
  These standards represent Cells 2 and 4 in Table 9-1. Outcome standards for
Cell 6 are commonly thought of in general terms such as decrease in inappropriate use of health services and improved patient and family well-being resulting from patient education.

TABLE 9-2.
ADULT PERFORMANCE LEVEL SKILLS AND KNOWLEDGE IN HEALTH

Goal: To understand the principles and practices that lead to good mental and physical health.
Major objective 1:   People should know where, when, and why to seek medical help. This means that they should
  A. recognize obvious signs of illness and know which requires professional attention.
  B. know the various types of medical facilities typically available in a community
  C. know how and why to follow medical instructions
  D. know how and why to communicate information about health problems to others
Major objective 2:   Individuals should know what personal habits promote good health. This means that they should
  A. know the basic principles of health maintenance
  B. know the basic principles of nutrition
  C. understand the relationship between drugs and health
Major objective 3:   Individuals should know how to apply principles of health to planning and raising a family. This means that they should
  A. understand the physical and psychologic influences of pregnancy and the need for proper prenatal care
  B. understand the importance of family planning and the effectiveness of various birth control practices
  C. know basic child-rearing practices
  D. understand the special health needs and concerns of adolescents
Major objective 4:   People should know how to deal with potential hazards and accidents. This means that they should
  A. recognize potential hazards
  B. know where and when to apply basic safety measures
  C. know when and how to apply first aid
  D. know how and whom to ask for help in emergencies

From Fagerberg, S., & Holyoak, O.J. The APL program in health and safety education. *Health Education*, 1978, *9(2)*, 8-9.

Outcome standards have become increasingly important with the pressure to justify activities and use of resources. Many standards represent *desired* outcomes; few seem to have been tested regarding their clinical attainability with particular target groups. A serious concern in such a situation is whether those standards constitute a misrepresentation, unless qualified as to groups that can be expected to meet them, measured by reasonably valid methods.

Outcome standards vary widely in specificity. One of the broadest is the adult performance level (APL) test which was developed by the Texas Department of Education.[3] The portions related to health may be seen in Table 9-2. They define skills and knowledge necessary for successful adult living in our society. The University of Texas project team that originally developed the tool conducted a national assessment that showed that nearly 20 percent of American adults cannot apply the skills they need to handle a variety of daily tasks.

At a more specific level are audit criteria in the area of patient knowledge and behavior for anesthesia nursing. This author chose to establish outcome criteria for specific anesthetic agents and/or techniques, as opposed to specific diagnoses or conditions (Table 9-3).[12]

TABLE 9-3.
EXAMPLE OF KNOWLEDGE OUTCOME CRITERIA
FOR SPECIFIC ANESTHETIC AGENTS AND/OR TECHNIQUES

Outcomes: General anesthesia—halothane
1. Patient verbalizes knowledge of side effects of halothane
    a. nausea and vomiting
    b. shivering
    c. temperature elevation
    d. jaundice
    e. severe headache
2. Patient verbalizes knowledge that side effects may occur after discharge from the hospital (e.g., jaundice, dark urine, nausea, and vomiting beyond the first 12 to 14 hours).
3. Patient verbalizes knowledge that side effects should be reported if they occur after discharge.

Outcomes: Intravenous infusion sites
1. Patient verbalizes an understanding for the changed IV sites that occur every 24 to 48 hours during prolonged IV therapy.

Outcomes: Spinal anesthesia—subarachnoid block
1. Patient verbalizes knowledge of side effects of SAB
    a. headache
    b. hypotension
    c. weakness of lower extremities several hours following return of motor and sensory function
    d. headache with diplopia
2. Patient verbalizes knowledge of what to do should side effects occur.

From Vail, J.D. Anesthesia nursing audit? yes! *Journal of the American Association of Nurse Anesthetists,* 1978, *46,* 127.

Other areas of care need to be concerned with behavioral outcomes over an extended period of time. An example is renal transplantation, for which criteria have been developed for two-week, one-month, three-month, and one-year intervals posttransplant (Table 9-4).[11] The particular recording form used with these criteria allows for indication of whether the criterion was met or not met, with comments and recommendations that might well take the form of exceptions to the criterion. This format seems excellent for trying out a set of criteria with a particular group of patients, to see whether they are attainable. They have the clear advantage of following the patient throughout a significant treatment interval, during which he needs to learn and make adaptations in his behavior.

Of considerable interest in developing outcome standards is the Wisconsin System for Nursing Quality Assurance, reported by Hover and Zimmer.[8] The system includes criteria, assessment, standards, and improvement of care. Each component is developed in order to implement the system. A major feature is that patient outcome criteria are limited to five per criteria set: (1) knowledge of illness and its treatment, (2) skills, (3) knowledge of medications, (4) adaptive behaviors, and (5) health or physiologic status. It was found that all patient outcomes can be subsumed within these five criteria, although not all of the criteria need to be included in each set.

TABLE 9-4.
SAMPLE OUTCOME CRITERIA FOR PATIENT BEHAVIOR AFTER KIDNEY TRANSPLANT*

Time Periods			
End of 2 Weeks	*End of 1 Month*	*End of 3 Months*	*End of 1 Year*
Patient and/or family contacts nurse/physician day or night when changes in physical status are recognized: a) decreased urine output, b) tenderness over kidney, c) blood in urine, d) general malaise, e) elevated temperature (more than 38.5 C), f) rapid weight gain (more than 2 lbs in one day or 4 lbs total in 7 days).	same	same	Patient continues to take correctly medications prescribed by his physician. Patient and/or family contacts nurse/physician when changes in physical status are recognized: a) abdomen pain, b) joint pain, c) pregnancy, d) visual changes.
Patient and/or family takes and records daily weight and temperature accurately and bring a complete record of the readings to each clinic visit.	same	same	
Patient and/or family demonstrates correct knowledge of prescribed medications by telling a) name of each drug, b) correct dosage and time patient takes medications, c) desired effect of each drug, d) side effects of medications.	same		
Patient and/or family asks for refills on medications as needed.	same		
Patient and/or family correctly demonstrates shunt, fistula, or surgical incision wound care.			
Patient and/or family verbalizes acceptable activity level of a) walking instead of running or jogging, b) no heavy lifting, c) no contact sports, d) no driving.	Patient and/or family verbalizes acceptable activity level of a) walking or running, b) no heavy lifting, c) no contact sports.		

(continued)

TABLE 9-4.

SAMPLE OUTCOME CRITERIA FOR PATIENT BEHAVIOR AFTER KIDNEY TRANSPLANT (Cont.)

Time Periods			
End of 2 Weeks	End of 1 Month	End of 3 Months	End of 1 Year
Patient and/or family easily discusses events following discharge with regard to acceptance of family members and peers.	same	same	Patient and/or family easily discusses continued adjustment to life as a kidney transplant recipient.
Patient and/or family easily discusses changes of physical appearance caused by immunosuppressive therapy: a) weight gain, b) hair loss, c) complexion changes, d) round cheeks, e) protruding abdomen, f)fat deposition over back.			The family easily discusses continued adjustment to life with a kidney recipient.
	Patient and/or family begins to verbalize plans with regard to future (career, school, and so on).	same	Patient is now working, going to school, or verbalizes acceptance of his life style.
	Patient and/or family correctly verbalizes knowledge of any prescribed dietary restrictions and principles of good nutrition.	same	
		Adult female reports obtaining regular gynecologic exams and pap smears.	
		Patient reports onset or change in menses.	
		Patient and/or family easily discusses their a) sexuality, b) concerns about sexual activity, c) and contraception.	

*Patient population: Adults and children discharged from the hospital following kidney transplant (all have functioning grafts). The acceptable degree of goal achievement is 100%.

Adapted from Sachs, B.L., & Hargrove, J.C. Patient outcome criteria: A tool for quality assurance. *Journal of the American Association of Nephrology Nurses and Technicians*, 1978, 5(1), 42–47.

To develop a new criteria set, a population must first be selected and assessment times determined. Assessment at several different points in time is desirable and can be accomplished by developing more than one criteria set for a single population or by using the same criteria set at different times.

Figure 9-2 shows sample outcome and charting guidelines. Note that for each skill, a list of all essential steps for correct performance should be constructed. The Wisconsin group is constructing an instrument for evaluation of knowledge of medications across all populations. Outcomes should be measurable by nurses and influenced at least in part by nursing care. Standards are not set until after the first evaluation has been completed, to add reality data to the judgment of what the criterion might be.

SPECULATION ON DEVELOPMENTS REGARDING QUALITY OF CARE IN PATIENT EDUCATION

It is likely that standards for patient education will shift rapidly if the present trend toward access by the client and the public to health information continues. Of course, the outcome of continuing consideration of third party reimbursement for this service will be a critical development.

New conceptual tools, such as a taxonomy of patient learning problems, banks of behavioral objectives, and further classification of the patient's overall ability to profit from patient education,[10] will be developed.

New patterns of patient involvement and their management will emerge. An example is development of a technology of self-measurement of daily disease progress and regimen effectiveness, such as with patients with cirrhosis.[4]

Tools for measuring outcomes of patient learning have been almost nonexistent. These will almost certainly develop in a standardized form, with good measurement characteristics (validity, reliability), which will greatly facilitate comparison of results within and between sites. More noninvasive measures, such as the measurement of compliance by chronic asthmatics with oral theophylline by analysis of saliva, are being developed.[2]

Areas in which there are apparently no standards, such as regulations defining what constitutes general "adequate directions for use" for a layman for a drug dispensed on prescription will probably be examined by regulatory agencies. The presumption that the directions provided by the physician are adequate may or may not remain tenable.[13]

SUMMARY

A simple structure within which to conceptualize criteria for quality of care for patient education has been presented. There are, no doubt, other structures that include more and other variables. Three different units of delivery—the

Population: Hospitalized patient 12 years of age or older who has received a kidney transplant.

Criteria I and III* may be measured via interview conducted by the audit team as part of a concurrent review. Criteria II, IV, and V should be assessed and recorded in the chart by unit staff. By the time of discharge, information as to the presence, absence, or extent of data should be included in the chart. This information may be retrieved on retrospective audit.

Criterion I: Knowledge of Illness and Treatment
    Prior to discharge, the patient should know the material included in "Home Care Information for Kidney Transplant Patients."

Criterion II: Skills
    If the steps listed under the skill are observed in the return demonstration, chart the skill as correctly demonstrated. If one or more steps are omitted or inaccurate, indicate this in the charting.
    Taking temperature
        1. Waiting 30 minutes after smoking, or eating or drinking hot or cold foods
        2. Shakes down thermometer till mercury is below 96 F
        3. Places thermometer under tongue
        4. Closes mouth
        5. Leaves thermometer in place for three full minutes
        6. Removes thermometer
        7. Holds at eye level in good light
        8. Reads mercury level
        9. Records reading
        10. Cleanses thermometer with warm water and soap
    Taking blood pressure
        1. Removes obstructive clothing from arm
        2. Sits in relaxed position with arm extended at heart level
        3. Wraps cuff evenly one inch above elbow with center of bladder over brachial artery
        4. Feels for pulse at elbow
        5. Positions gauge so it can be read easily
        6. Closes valve on bulb
        7. Pumps bulb until the gauge reads 20-30 mm Hg above usual systolic reading
        8. Opens valve slowly 2-3 mm Hg/sec
        9. Notes point at which tapping sound is first heard
        10. Notes point at which tapping sound ceases
        11. Records blood pressure reading

Criterion IV: Adaptive Behaviors
    Patient maintains daily intake and output records, and own medication records

Criterion V: Health and Physiologic Status
    At time of discharge, the chart should include
        1. Description of urine to include presence or absence of clearness, mucus, sediment, blood
        2. Presence or absence of edema
        3. Description of wound to include presence or absence of dryness, swelling, discoloration, healing
        4. Presence/absence of oral herpes, glossitis, stomatitis, diarrhea, constipation, gastric burning or pain, nausea or vomiting

Note: Criterion III is Knowledge of Medications. An instrument is being developed to measure this knowledge across all populations.

Figure 9-2.
Sample outcome and charting guidelines. (From Hover, J., & Zimmer, M. J. Nursing quality assurance: The Wisconsin system. *Nursing Outlook,* April, 1978, 26(4):242-248. Copyright © 1978, American Journal of Nursing Company. Reproduced with permission from *Nursing Outlook.*)

individual patient, the program, and the delivery system—are considered since each presents particular problems for quality of patient education.

While outcome (change in patient behavior) standards are still being developed, both they and process standards can play an important role. A major task now is to study and document the degree to which process and outcome standards are related for particular conditions and patients.

REFERENCES

1. Delano, B. G., & Friedman, E. A. Successful home hemodialysis in the ghetto. *Dialysis and Transplantation,* 1977, *6,* 64–73.
2. Eney, R. D., & Goldstein, E. O. Compliance of chronic asthmatics with oral administration as measured by serum and salivary levels. *Pediatrics,* 1976, *57,* 513–517.
3. Fagerberg, S., & Holyoak, O. J. APL program in health and safety education. *Health Education,* 1978, *9(2),* 8–9.
4 Goldstein, M. K., Stein, G. H., Smolen, D. M., & Perlini, W. S. Bio-behavioral monitoring: A method for remote health measurement. *Archives of Physical Medicine Rehabilitation,* 1976, *57,* 253–258.
5. Green, L. W. Toward cost-benefit evaluations of health education: Some concepts, methods and examples. *Health Education Monographs,* 1974, *2* (Suppl.), 36–64.
6. Green, L. W., & Figa-Talamance, I. Suggested designs for evaluation of patient education programs. *Health Education Monographs,* 1974, *2,* 54–71.
7. Hirsh, H. L. Informed consent—fact or fiction? *Journal of Legal Medicine,* 1977, *5,* 25–27.
8. Hover, J., & Zimmer, M. J. Nursing quality assurance: the Wisconsin system. *Nursing Outlook,* 1978, *16,* 242–248.
9. Katz, H., & Clancy, R. R. Accuracy of a home throat culture program: A study of parent participation of health care. *Pediatrics,* 1974, *53,* 687–691.
10. Redman, B. K. *The process of patient teaching in nursing,* 3rd ed. St. Louis, Mosby, 1976.
11. Sachs, B. L., & Hargrove, J. C. Patient outcome criteria: a tool for quality assurance. *Journal of the American Association of Nephrology Nurses and Technicians,* 1978, *5,* 41–48.
12. Vail, J. D. Anesthesia nursing audit? Yes! *Journal of the American Association of Nurse Anesthetists,* 1978, *46,* 125–129.
13. Valentino, J. G. An analysis of the regulatory and legal aspects of patient package inserts. *Journal of the American Pharmaceutical Association,* 1977, *17,* 688–691.

10

PREPARING NURSES TO TEACH

A number of elements presumably determine how patient education is practiced. One such element is the delivery system, the degree to which it makes teaching possible and is supportive of its delivery. This element is addressed in another book (*Patterns for Distribution*) in this series and might be said to reflect (probably with a cultural lag) general societal support and demand for the practice. A second element is the educational and experiential preparation of nurses to deliver this service. Both preservice and inservice preparation are important, especially since the quality of such preparation is not known and is likely to have been variable over the years and among schools of nursing.

What we now view as the "nursing model" is relatively recent and represents a reemphasis on psychosocial care and perhaps a different integration of it with other elements of nursing practice. What one can expect is considerable variability in nurses' ability to teach patients and in their perceptions of whether and how it is an element of nursing practice.

One of the most persistent difficulties in the development of this field is the lack of clarity about what teaching behaviors are important for nurses to learn. The field of education has also had considerable difficulty with this matter, since there are tremendous pressures to hold teachers and schools accountable for student growth. Most process-product studies of teacher behavior (studies of the relationship between teaching and the long-term goal) have failed to identify specific behaviors that consistently and predictably affect student learning in elementary schools. Some researchers believe that no research base exists to provide direction for the selection of competencies that are to be mastered in teacher education programs.[2]

Although this author knows of no such studies in patient or health education done in health settings, one would assume that the same general state of knowledge about teaching process and learning product would hold. Even given this doubtfulness, nurses must have diagnostic or assessment skills to recognize need for behavior change, to be able to deliver teaching within a nursing role, and to be able to evaluate the client outcome. What is unclear is whether there is one exact set of nurse/teacher behaviors that will best yield the patient outcomes. This means that as in other areas of nursing, the teaching component may be viewed in large part as an art and that specific process behaviors (such as a specific interpersonal style or using the teaching process in exact sequential order) should not be required. It is, however, of considerable use to teach nurses varieties of teaching strategies which they can then use in their practice.

ELEMENTS OF A GOOD INSTRUCTIONAL PROGRAM IN PATIENT EDUCATION FOR NURSES

There are some general elements that appear useful for preparing nurses to do patient education in both pre- and inservice preparation.

PROFICIENCY IN KNOWLEDGE AND SKILL

Cognitive knowledge about how people learn is important but clearly not sufficient to teach patients. It is, however, probably the easiest to learn inexpensively, as from reading a book. Given the present state of its scientific accuracy, it cannot be expected to comprehensively direct practice. There may well be practical instances which no known theory of learning or teaching explains or to which two different theories give conflicting directions. Knowledge about teaching and learning can provide general direction for the process of teaching, information about some learning processes, and strategies that have been useful in getting learning to occur.

Skill in delivering patient education may not be highly correlated with knowledge about teaching and learning. It also probably represents a heterogeneous group of skills, some of which have to do with picking up and capitalizing on the readiness skills of patients, relating to patients in a way that makes them want to learn, and to provide instructional material. Organizational skills, such as negotiating with others who care for the patient, make instruction available.

Another essential component is accurate information and understanding of the material the patient is to learn, and skill in those skills he is to develop. Obviously, lack of this knowledge and skill is serious and probably not uncommon. Simply working in a unit caring for patients with particular difficulties does not insure this adequate knowledge and skill base. Several delivery modes have been developed to minimize this problem, such as for nurses on a medical-surgical unit, who care for patients with different problems, each specializing in having the content knowledge necessary to teach one of these groups of patients.

PRACTICE TIME

Partly because the skills and knowledge base necessary to teach are so imperfectly known, practice to the level of confidence and competence in obtaining desirable patient outcomes is essential. These experiences force the nurse to devise his or her own set of strategies and decision points based on actual patient behavior. It is the author's opinion that this element in the preparation of nurses to teach is the least available, particularly if one includes the necessary supervision and feedback that are essential to making the practice educational for the nurse.

FEEDBACK

Consistent with the position taken earlier, the feedback to the nurse on how he or she did in teaching patients should be focused on ability to create patient outcomes within ethical means and on alternate possible interpretations of patient behavior and strategies to use. The feedback is then not so much prescriptive of one particular process but broadening in developing a range of skills. Videotaped feedback is useful because it provides a fuller range (including nonverbal) of information and a reality that is often motivating to the nurse. Audits can be used as feedback as well as a focus for group motivation in improving this area of practice.

A couple of examples of how these elements are put together in courses are available in the literature.[1,4]

PREPARATION FOR PATIENT EDUCATION IN PRESERVICE CURRICULUM FRAMEWORKS

Staff development in a service setting tends to be oriented to competencies that will be used on the job. Preservice education for nurses has been undergoing considerable ferment with curriculum frameworks. How does this activity affect preparation for patient education?

In general, the new frameworks have aimed to (1) more accurately portray the nursing model rather than the old medical model curriculums, and (2) integrate the numerous theoretical and practice strands that had accumulated into a more manageable structure. Reflecting these two purposes, in many new curricula faculty have, for example, chosen to focus on the nursing process as it assists man's adaptation in health and illness.

Adequate preparation for patient education can be done in a variety of curriculum models, as long as the instructional elements outlined in the previous section are available. Several problems in making these elements available have not been uncommon:

1. Some curricula have not adequately interrelated the patient needs and nursing skills or do not have a balance between them in the instructional program. This can mean that the student learns a lot about patient needs and not much about nursing intervention or vice versa, or learns them separately instead of what and how patient needs can be addressed with regard to patient education.
2. The new integrated conceptual framework does not have a "home" for patient education or it is so thoroughly "integrated" that the student does not

develop skills of any depth. Perhaps the most obvious "home" for patient education is helping relationships, although information about how man learns can be included in information about adaptation. However, the realm of helping relationships often is a very confused jumble of "interpersonal relationships, communication, psychiatric nursing, patient support," and so on. What is unclear is how all these overlap, interrelate, or are separate. The author's attempt at such clarification has been developed in Chapter 7.

3. Most critical is the availability of good clinical experience in patient education. Primarily, this depends on adequate faculty skill in patient education and on availability of clinical facilities with these kinds of learning experiences. It is possible, however, for the curriculum structure to be so diffuse or confused in its focus that clinical experiences are similarly unfocused. Another possible misfortune is that there are so many foci for the available clinical hours that some of them get short shrift.

It is, then, possible to do a creditable job of preparing nurses to teach, in a variety of curricular patterns. As usual, it is likely to be the clarity of purpose and skills of the faculty that become the critical variables.

LEVELS OF PATIENT EDUCATION SKILL IN THE NURSING DEGREE STRUCTURES

The practice of patient education clearly offers variability in levels of difficulty and of skill required. Perhaps least difficult are patients with good ability to learn independently, who are not being asked to make multiple life changes, who are eager to cooperate, who have conditions for which teaching is accepted as useful, with fairly standardized easy-to-understand content, taught in a supportive setting. Anything contrary to these will often indicate problems.

Nurses also need program development and evaluation skills as well as administrative skills. Master's curricula rarely have a comprehensive conceptual framework but rather present the conceptual focus of the area of specialization (parent-child nursing, psychiatric-mental health nursing, and so on). Whether much focus is given to patient education is likely to be highly variable. The conceptual foci of the specialties usually do not require it, although a tradition of use of patient education in a field (such as parent-child nursing) may affect its inclusion.

As is not uncommon, there are likely to be gaps among skills that might be provided in a baccalaureate program, the demands of the jobs in which any nurse finds him- or herself, and the skills provided in a Master's program.

PREPARATION FOR PATIENT EDUCATION IN THE NURSE PRACTITIONER ROLE

Skill in patient education should be a prerequisite for practice in this role. Primary care, which is where many nurse practitioners work, requires these skills developed to a high level in order to deal quite independently with resistant patients, those whose health problems and social situations do not support changed behavior, and others with similar difficulties. The practitioner's practice may well focus the content that he or she will need to teach patients and the difficulties of the behavioral tasks they must master. The elements of skill, knowledge, and clinical practice as outlined earlier in the chapter are applicable.

SKILLS FOR THE SPECIALIST EDUCATOR ROLE

Perhaps the oldest and best developed example of the specialist is the diabetes educator. The field has an organization and a journal. Recognition of the important role education plays in the care of the patient with diabetes has existed for at least 50 years. It is probable that the work in diabetes education over a period of time has played a significant part in the current impetus for expanded patient education and hospital-based health education programs in the United States.[5]

This person has educational responsibilities over and above those of other members of the health care team, and skills are more advanced as well. The task requires someone who is moderately sophisticated in diabetes management, and who is knowledgeable about the jobs of the health care team and operations of the clinic or inpatient service. The person has to be able to understand fairly complex material and to be able to translate this into simple everyday sentences if necessary. The task requires knowledge of patients' problems and how they can be solved, and the problems diabetes poses as a medical condition. The usual instructional tasks include explaining diabetes; providing dietary instruction; teaching urine testing; instructing the patient and family in administration of insulin when appropriate; explaining use of oral hypoglycemic agents when appropriate, acute and other complications, and the role of exercise; instructing the patient in proper foot care, personal hygiene, and preventive measures; counseling the patient about adapting his present living pattern to diabetes; and introducing the patient to the continuing care system. But also most important for this kind of patient is focus on motivational incentives and social support systems. Ongoing staff education is also often required of the diabetes educator, so that congruent instruction is given by staff to patients.[5]

The existence of diabetes educators means that the educational responsibilities and functions have grown to such proportions that someone must devote full time to them. Similar patterns are occurring in the cardiovascular, respiratory, arthritis, parenting, and perhaps other fields. This author knows of no formal educational programs that specifically focus on preparation for this role, although more general programs may allow such focus by individual student election. In general, such specialist positions are filled by nurses who have by long clinical practice and diligent study with co-workers obtained many of the skills needed.

TABLE 10-1.
HOSPITAL-BASED CONSUMER HEALTH EDUCATION COORDINATORS*
JOB DESCRIPTION AND SKILLS

Job Description: The coordinator of patient and community health education shall be responsible for carrying out some or all of the following functions within the setting of the health care facility and its surrounding community.

A.   Planning and Administration of Health Education Programs
   1. Identifying and evaluating health education needs within the hospital[†] by means of cooperative efforts between department personnel.
   2. Identifying and evaluating health education needs within the hospital's community or service area by means of cooperative efforts with community agencies and groups.
   3. Working with other hospital and community people to establish priorities for patient and community health education program development.
   4. Planning and administering consumer health education programs such that they include an accurate statement of need, a set of measurable objectives, a definitive course outline, specific teaching, methodologies, and integrated, ongoing evaluations.
   5. Preparing and administering evaluation methodologies for consumer health education programs in the hospital and community.
   6. Supervising personnel such as health counselors, patient teachers, out-reach workers, students, volunteers, and secretaries.
   7. Establishing and maintaining liaison between the hospital and representatives of public, private, and voluntary agencies, and consumer groups for purposes of health education program planning.
   8. Establishing and reporting to appropriate hospital and community advisory committees for advisement and approval of the patient and community health education programs.
   9. Assisting in the creation, identification, and review of teaching materials necessary for implementing health education programs (printed and/or audiovisual).
   10. Identifying, organizing, and supervising the necessary manpower to teach health education programs in the hospital and surrounding communities. This includes using the resources of such departments as inservice, medical education, nursing, outpatient, social service, dietary, volunteers, pharmacy, etc.
   11. Assisting in staff development programs that provide and/or improve the skills of professionals teaching health education programs to patients and community lay persons.
   12. Preparing and submitting health education program budgets to the appropriate administrative personnel.
   13. Creating, organizing, and maintaining a record system relevant and useful for the hospital's education programs.
   14. Preparing and seeking approval for educational program standards to meet third party reimbursement criteria.

B.   General Administration and Communications
   1. Establishing vertical lines of communication in order to carry suggestions to, and recommendations from, the hospital management team regarding the integration of health education into health care delivery.

(continued)

*Hereafter the term "consumer health education coordinator" will be shortened to "coordinator."
†The term "hospital" is being used to include the health centers and health maintenance organizations.

From *Training Hospital-Based Health Education Coordinates: A Report of a Pilot Curriculum.* Piscataway, New Jersey, College of Medicine and Dentistry of New Jersey, Office of Consumer Health Education, April, 1977. This project was supported by a grant from the New Jersey Regional Medical Program Inc.

TABLE 10-1
HOSPITAL-BASED CONSUMER HEALTH EDUCATION COORDINATORS
JOB DESCRIPTION AND SKILLS (Cont.)

---

2. Relating current and future health education plans to the overall hospital budget. Preparing and submitting a health education department or program budget to the appropriate administrative personnel. Working with hospital financial personnel with regard to third party reimbursement and long-term financial viability of the hospital's health education program.
3. Conducting ongoing evaluation of the overall health education program of the hospital.
4. Working with the public relations and other hospital departments to develop commitment and support for the health education programs within the hospital and community.
5. Providing consultation services for the hospital and community agencies regarding health education programming.
6. Representing and communicating the hospital's policies on health education at community, state, and national levels.
7. Maintaining liaison with the Office of Consumer Health Education or another source for purposes of technical assistance, evaluation, and input at the national level.

Skills: Each of the functions previously listed for coordinators requires one or more specialized skills. These skills can be obtained through either academic and/or professional work experience. Below is a list of the skills the Office of Consumer Health Education has identified as essential to the functioning of consumer health education coordinators.
1. Administration and supervision.
2. Program planning, budgeting, and evaluation.
3. Diagnosis of community health and health education needs.
4. Community organization and development.
5. Working knowledge of organizational and interorganizational development within the hospital and community.
6. Working knowledge of how to identify, utilize, and manage human, fiscal, and material resources (materials include pamphlets, brochures, audiovisuals).
7. Working knowledge of teaching and learning principles for adults and children.
8. Working knowledge of interpersonal, group, and written communication processes.
9. Working knowledge of health education and behavioral science principles.
10. Working knowledge of the health care system.
11. Working knowledge of research methodology in health and health education.

Qualifications:
1. Academic preparation—Master's degree preferred in health or health related field. A minimum of a baccaluareate in health or a health related field or an R.N. received from a three-year diploma school.
2. Professional experience—A minimum of two years of professional health or health related experience preferred. Administrative and managerial experience should be part of this professional experience.
3. Possible professional background include: Nursing, pharmacy, allied health, behavioral sciences, education, health education, social work, nutrition, and so forth.

THE NEW JERSEY PROJECT TO TRAIN HOSPITAL-BASED CONSUMER HEALTH EDUCATION COORDINATORS[6]

In 1972 and 1973, the College of Medicine and Dentistry of New Jersey's consumer health education program began. The associated hospitals and community health centers undertook long and sometimes futile searches for qualified individuals to head their programs. The college then piloted a program to train a group of health professionals for positions that were primarily administrative. Their duties included overseeing planning, implementation, and evaluation of patient and community health education programs. The job description and skills for this program appear in Table 10-1. (See pages 91–92.)

TOOL FOR DESCRIPTION OF LEVEL OF USE OF THE INNOVATION

Incorporation of teaching into nursing practice can constitute an innovation. So, also, can use of a particular program or approach with patients, the introduction of a new course on patient education, or helping relationships in a curriculum. A general scale for describing how well an innovation is employed could be of considerable use in such situations. It is based on the notion that

TABLE 10-2.
SCALE POINT DEFINITIONS OF THE LEVELS OF USE OF THE INNOVATION

Level	Definition
Level 0	*Non-use:* State in which the user has little or no knowledge of the innovation, no involvement with the innovation, and is doing nothing toward becoming involved.
Level I	*Orientation:* State in which the user has recently acquired or is acquiring information about the innovation and/or has recently explored or is exploring its value orientation and its demands upon user and user system.
Level II	*Preparation:* State in which the user is preparing for first use of the innovation.
Level III	*Mechanical use:* State in which the user focuses on the short-term, day-to-day use of the innovation with little time for reflection. Changes in use are made more to meet user needs than client needs. The user is primarily engaged in a stepwise attempt to master the tasks required to use the innovation, often resulting in disjointed and superficial use.
Level IVA	*Routine:* Use of the innovation is stabilized. Few if any changes are being made in ongoing use. Little preparation or thought is being given to improving innovation use or its consequences.
Level IVB	*Refinement:* State in which the user varies the use of the innovation to increase the impact on clients within immediate sphere of influence. Variations are based on knowledge of both short- and long-term consequences for clients.
Level V	*Integration:* State in which the user is combining own efforts to use the innovation with related activities of colleagues to achieve a collective impact on clients within their common sphere of influence.
Level VI	*Renewal:* State in which the user reevaluates the quality of use of the innovation, seeks major modifications of or alternatives to present innovation to achieve increased impact on clients, examines new developments in the field, and explores new goals for self and the system.

From Hall et al. Levels of use of the innovation: A framework for analyzing innovation adoption. *Journal of Teacher Education*, 1975, *26(1)*, 53–56.

growth in quality of use of an innovation by most individuals is developmental and is not likely to be completed until several cycles of use, and that this development may need to be assisted. This tool and its use are described more fully in the original source.[3] Through interviews with people who are to be implementing the innovation, and other data sources, individuals are classified as to level, and strategies are planned to further assist implementation of the innovation (Table 10-2).

SUMMARY

Material from a training project and a tool to check degree to which nurses are incorporating teaching into their practice or into a curriculum have been presented. Such materials are rare; yet some degree of preparation for the patient education role is occurring in preservice, inservice, and continuing education programs. Certain elements of preparation seem likely to be necessary: these include strong focus on confidence in delivery skills as well as ability to independently think through the processes of teaching and learning.

REFERENCES

1. Chapman, J. J. Microteaching: How students learn group patient education skills. *Nurse Educator*, 1978, *3*, 13–16.
2. Good, T. L., Biddle, B. J., & Brophy, J. E. *Teachers make a difference*. New York: Holt, 1975.
3. Hall, G. E., Loucks, S., Rutherford, W., & Newlove, B. Levels of use of the innovation: A framework for analyzing innovation adoption. *Journal of Teacher Education*, 1975, *26(1)*, 52–56.
4. Jenny, J. Patient teaching as a curriculum thread. *The Canadian Nurse*, 1978, *74*, 28–29.
5. Simonds, S. K. Competency-based training for the diabetes educator. *The Diabetes Educator*, 1978, *4(1)*, 5–10.
6. *Training hospital-based health education coordinators: A report of a pilot curriculum*. Piscataway, New Jersey, College of Medicine and Dentistry of New Jersey, Office of Consumer Health Education, 1977. This project was supported by a grant from the New Jersey Regional Medical Program, Inc.

11

EMERGING POLICY, THEORY, AND RESEARCH ISSUES FOR PATIENT EDUCATION

An understanding of broad-based issues in a field assists in obtaining perspective about the level of present practice and what forces will likely affect it in the next few years. Issues in patient education are multiple and include limitations in basic theory and research, decisions about the kind of programming that should be done in the field, about who will direct practice, and about systems for practice, development of the knowledge base, and, just barely beginning, on individualization of instruction. Some of these issues and directions are selected for discussion in this chapter.

WHO MAKES DECISIONS ABOUT PATIENT EDUCATION?

Consumer pressures will continue. Perhaps equally great pressures will come from health professionals who wish to be able to practice patient education professionally. Many, including health educators, feel they function as behavior change technicians. Programs generally take their essential content from physicians and translate that content into behavior-change strategies. Health education has been a highly process-oriented profession, which is congruent with the expectation that others will concern themselves with *what* should be changed.[3]

This author believes clarification about professional prerogatives will be slow and that although change will come in many ways, probably the most common way will be negotiation for responsibility for programs, which will then become a more permanent delegation.

BROAD PROGRAMMING TOPICS

Predominant program topics now seem to be in particular chronic illnesses, in reduction of certain risk behaviors such as smoking, and controlling obesity and hypertension. Such topics are perhaps popular because they can show immediate cost containment and because for chronic illness there is not much alternative to people managing much of their own care.

One would hope that in addition to careful expansion, patient education would also emphasize creative new programming. Of special interest to nurses is that oriented toward health. Wellness is often seen to include the development of competence including ability to master one's own self and one's life situation including responsibility for one's own health.[4]

An example of such a health-promoting group is the parent-infant support group which is conducted during the first months of the infant's life. The group began in Washington, D. C., in 1973 because of concern that not much attention was being paid to the problem of how to promote the primary needs of the average new parent and the healthy infant. The groups consisted of 8 to 10 mothers with their infants and a leader, working in a teaching-learning, not a therapy, relationship, in something like an extended family environment where mothers could feel support in their relationships with their infants. The challenge was to actively create a new life-style for the family, which met the needs of the parents and the baby. The need seemed to be greatest when the infant was newborn to four months of age, for it is then that the mother feels most isolated emotionally and physically.[13]

Further examples of what might be thought of as innovative programming arise because many societies in the world have reached or are reaching their absorptive capacity to further provide monies for the establishment of new or expanded service systems. For care of the elderly, linkages between families and service bureaucracies might be strengthened and better articulated so that the combination more efficiently provides what the elderly need.[9] Involved in such alterations would be instruction of families in care of their elderly and in use of the service bureaucracies. Some feel that a better balance needs to be attained between professional and lay services, each doing what it can do best.

INDIVIDUALIZATION OF INSTRUCTION

It is obvious that not everyone benefits from the same instruction. General rules for these differences exist and have been addressed throughout this text but are very rough and imprecise and often provide minimal direction for how to help a particular patient to learn.

So, also, research about individual differences in bases for behavior and in response to instruction is barely beginning, and much of it cannot yet be considered reliable as a basis for instruction. To make things more complex, often individuality for a particular health action involves interaction of several proclivities and environmental cues. And often, a study that shows differences in groups of people is not designed to elucidate why these differences occur, how generalizable they are, and whether the logical interventions they propose actually work.

Understanding that such differences exist and what might be potent differences in an area of behavior is still useful, since it provides an explanation for why an intervention did not work and a notion of how it might be altered to work better.

EXPLAINING HEALTH BEHAVIOR DIFFERENCES

That people have different patterns of response to health situations and stimuli is obvious. What those patterns are, how stable they are, and how well they explain the individual behavior are being studied. Single studies are cited in several areas to give the reader a notion of a variety of ways in which individualization is being conceptualized.

Breast Cancer Detection

In trying to understand why some women fail to participate in preventive and early detection screening programs for breast cancer while others do not, variables such as anxiety; knowledge of and personal experience with cancer; image of physician attitudes, norms, and supports; and involvement in the world of illness and medicine were examined in one study.[1]

The conclusion of the study was a fourfold typology of women, which attempted to explain the circumstances under which these different types would likely voluntarily take part in breast cancer examination. The "conformist" type was highly sensitive to conformity to the norms of her reference groups. She is not likely to take independent initiative and would likely respond primarily to institutionalized mechanisms and social pressures, followed by reinforcement until the behavior was ritualized.

The "rational, goal-directed" woman was the type toward whom the traditional cancer education program has been aimed, with its focus on rational self-interest and knowledge of symptoms and benefits. She is inner-directed and tends to evaluate and rank alternative behavior patterns in terms of their consistency with consciously defined goals. She is likely to have a relatively high educational background.

The "complacent-stoic" woman has a positive image of the medical institution, does not see herself as less susceptible than others, has low anxiety, and is in general hard to budge. A clear symptom, upsetting her usual ability to function, will move her to action, but it would have to be quite clear. This type may best respond to stress on self-examination. Discovery of a symptom may constitute a sufficient disturbance of homeostasis to lead to action.

Finally, the "ambivalent-anxious" type is generally fearful of what preventive actions may find and her self-image is ambivalent and shifting. Her pattern is one of instability and unpredictability, with neither a sense of mastery and stable adaptation to her world nor a sense of submission, which can be no less stably adaptive. For her, locating cancer examination in the context of general examinations may be appropriate.[1]

While this research is quite preliminary, it does illustrate the notion of different patterns of resistance resources, patterns of behavior that follow, and suggested intervention methods that are different but aimed at each particular pattern.

Effectiveness of Contraception

Several further examples are instructive. Approached from the point of view of the field of communication, one study focused on differences in such patterns between groups of women who consistently succeeded in preventing pregnancy, and another who failed repeatedly. Both groups had contraceptive information and devices and were from similar social backgrounds. Women who succeeded in contraception excelled in their general competence as communicators, were significantly higher in self-esteem, more frank and direct, and disclosed at a significantly higher rate than did the ineffective contraceptor groups.[5] These findings join other findings regarding women who were effective and ineffective at contraception, some focusing on relationship between partners and some on beliefs about vulnerability to pregnancy. The task of research, eventually to be used in practice, is to describe as many of these differences as can be found with accurate measurements and determine how they interact with particular groups in particular situations, and how one can reliably determine these differences in clinical practice so as to select interventions that will be effective with a particular combination of individual differences.

Diabetics

A personality variable of particular interest recently has been locus of control (a continuum from external to internal) where an internal person believes that he or she can affect his or her world. The superiority of the internal in respect to information acquisition and utilization has been replicated using a variety of tasks. Also, internals are less open to influence than are externals. One study of this variable with diabetics verified that internals knew more about diabetes than did externals. Indeed, there has been a consistent tendency in locus of control literature to assume that the internal's tendency to seek information will usually result in superiority of self-management. This study does not support this tendency and hypothesizes that because some diabetics cannot be completely controlled with the information available to medicine about the disease and its treatment, the internal may encounter information that is either too vague to be of much help or is actually misleading. With his typical response ineffective (information does not produce control) and his personality that will not allow him to comply passively, he reacts against the situation and gives up some of the control he originally exercised. The external is not interested in control; instead, he follows what is for him the normal course of compliance with authority, which is seeing the physician and following the regimen. This is the more adaptive set of responses than is that of the internal.[7]

Note that in this situation where information is invalid or cannot produce control, the internal's usual ways of coping create a disadvantage. One would assume that he could be taught other coping strategies. Literature on locus of control in health situations has not yet produced consistent results and should be expected to vary with the elements of the situation as the example above indicates.

Asthmatics

A final example of individualization of response comes from a study done of management of asthma in a population whose disease is severe and intractable.[6] During treatment, neither the objective medical severity of the patient's asthma as determined by spirometric pulmonary function measurements and the physician's judgment about the severity of the asthma, nor whether he was prescribed maintenance oral corticosteroids at discharge, adequately predicted rate of rehospitalization after discharge. High panic-fear personality types did have higher rehospitalization rates. This type seems to exaggerate subjective symptoms as though they lack adaptive ways to deal with the illness and thus respond to airway obstruction with feelings of helplessness and panic. These patients seem to engage in a behavioral cycle that disrupts their medical program. On experiencing breathing difficulties, they "panic" and attempt to alleviate the difficulties by overmedicating. Upon stabilizing their asthma, they then focus on the potential side effects of their medical regimen and try to reduce this risk by undermedicating. This pattern finally results in rehospitalization, also affected by the psychophysiologic effects on breathing.

Low panic-fear patients show a different but equally maladaptive response style. It is known that they are discharged from treatment earlier than others and receive less intensive medication despite similarities in pulmonary function measurements. They are deniers, who unrealistically minimize their physical discomfort, not responding to increased airway obstruction by appropriately increasing distress-related treatments. They may allow an asthmatic attack to progress to the point that treatment short of rehospitalization is insufficient to control the attack.

Intervention presumably should be aimed at enhancing the high panic-fear patient's perceived personal control over and his understanding of the predictable aspects of his illness. For low panic-fear patients, efforts are needed to reduce the patient's denial, to enhance his internal awareness of increased breathing problems, and to follow the medical regimen even when feeling well.[6] Well-tested interventions to achieve these goals with these patients need to be verified and developed.

EXPLAINING INTERVENTION FAILURES

Some consideration of individual differences comes after intervention programs are examined and found to be disappointing.

Smoking Cessation

One author[2] believes achieving abstinence from smoking may be unrelated to maintaining abstinence, and that much more attention has been directed to attaining than to maintaining. This study focused on one element of individual difference, that of timing of the teaching designed to change the person's attitude toward smoking. Whenever the individual subject first becomes ready for change, his motivation is maximal and the treatment should be given.

Looking at smoking cessation more broadly, other authors comment on difficulties in this field with their major argument relating to lack of clarity in the field of individual differences.[10] Most self-help, stop-smoking products provide little in the way of structure beyond the first brief period off cigarettes. Most clinics, on the other hand, involve the smoker in an intensive time-consuming concentrated program that too often ends while the neonate ex-smoker is just beginning to grapple with withdrawal symptoms. Help for the phase of achieving abstinence is available only in small doses or in large doses; there appears to be no in between. The American Health Foundation has developed an initial smoking history questionnaire and a follow-up questionnaire to try to predict probable success at specific levels of intervention. In all probability, a hierarchical series of programs will be called for.[10]

CONCEPTUAL APPROACH TO PATIENT CARE RESEARCH CONGRUENT WITH CLINICAL PRACTICE ROLE

As has been indicated previously, much of the research base for patient education has been borrowed from school education, with little known about how well it can be transferred. In addition, psychosocial interventions in patient care often contain several elements, some or all of which may be seen as teaching. And since people's definitions of teaching vary widely, elements of the intervention need to be specified. For example, one series of studies focused on reduction of situationally derived psychologic distress from hospital stress by a deliberative intervention that included cognitive structuring, expression of emotions, and active participation by patients with feedback.[12]

In addition, clinical research has had its own problems in adaptation of research models from other fields. In particular, there were questions about sample size, possible bias if nurse clinicians combined research with clinical practice, precision of definition of the independent variable especially for replication. Development of the CLEM (Clinical Experimental Method) provides a conceptual and operational model that deals with these issues. This approach has been used in a series of small sample investigations of the deliberative intervention as described above, with patients in labor and delivery, pediatric surgery, and postsurgical pain. Viewed as a whole, the studies provided strong evidence that many hospital activities produce high levels of psychosocial stress in patients, that the resulting patient distress can be greatly reduced through deliberative interaction between patients and clinicians, and that reduction in patient distress can greatly enhance the effectiveness of medical interventions and can promote rapid recovery. They suggest that psychosocial prophylaxis of stress may have broad ramifications for the improvement of hospital-based inpatient care.[12]

CLEM provides methods for initial exploration of hypotheses including those arising from clinical experience, in which one discovers a new way of handling a problem that seems to get better results than the old way. The process allows for small samples of patients with one or two nurse clinicians conducting the research, using measures that are objective, blind, or both; these can be collected over an extended period of time. The first experiments testing a theory often operationalize the independent variable in broad terms; replication tests approximately the same theory in an approximately equivalent manner. If results are in the same direction and not grossly different in magnitude, they are interpreted as consistent. Once exploratory experiments have indicated general areas in which further structuring of research procedures is required and how it can best be accomplished, replications that are operationally precise can be designed. Types of subjects for whom the experimental intervention is found to be unsuccessful can be eliminated from the sample, and the sample size increased to obtain greater precision in the evaluation of treatment effects. Aspects of the experimental intervention that seem ineffective or too difficult to manipulate can be dropped or manipulated in a different way. Those aspects that seem crucial can be made part of an explicit procedures list. Theoretically distinct components of the intervention can be manipulated separately. Dependent variable measures found to be unreliable, insensitive, or redundant can be dropped or modified, and the remaining variables measured with increased care and precision. Additional dependent variables can be added, and as the knowledge base provided by initial experimentation increases, larger scale replication of greater complexity and precision can be designed.[12]

The full consideration of articulation of research with the clinical role makes the model a prime tool for development of a sounder research base for patient education practice.

Development of systematic research in health education indeed has a high priority. What work has been done, with the exception of the Health Belief Model, is generally not developed in a programmatic way over a period of time so as to afford a systematic way of dealing with the many variables and then moving on.[11]

PRIORITY ON DEVELOPMENT OF A SYSTEM

As they are currently provided, health education services are based in a multitude of agencies and institutional arrangements at local, state, and national levels. Each of these has a unique history of voluntary or governmental sponsorship and program development and usually does not have health education as a solitary objective. Delivery settings can be categorized as follows:

1. Educational institutions (public and private schools, colleges and universities)
2. Health organizations (voluntary health agencies, health departments, and other official agencies)
3. Health care facilities (hospitals, HMOs, clinics, ambulatory care centers)
4. Media organizations (television, radio, newspaper)
5. Employment settings (business and industry)[11]

In each of these delivery settings, each institution, agency, or facility has a delivery system of its own, functioning more or less loosely. The particular missions of each in relation to the broad, generally accepted goals for national health and the individual characteristics of their institutional arrangements make them not nearly so compatible as collaborators in a comprehensive health education delivery system as one might ideally hope.[11]

Comprehensiveness as a systems goal needs further definition. Examples of lack of comprehensiveness and continuity are very easy to find. Pless,[8] who has long had an interest in the delivery of health services to handicapped children and their families, first studied children with meningomyelocele and subsequently a group with chronic arthropathies. Parents' perceptions suggested a pattern whereby basic care was either divided or duplicated between specialists and primary physicians. There may be no clear understanding about which party is to assume the major responsibility for each facet of care. But in addition, many of the supportive aspects of care were found to be neglected in a high proportion of families. One major gap was in the area of "advice." Questions in this category dealt with discipline, adjustment to handicap, problems associated with schooling, and discussions with parents about the "total child." Another deficiency was in planning for the future and a third failure was not providing genetic counseling, although a number of parents had questions about whether their other or future children could get the disease.

SUMMARY

In summary, the issues facing patient and health education are broad and basic. They include questions about societal priorities and about professional development of the research base for the field and about improvements in practice and delivery.

REFERENCES

1. Antonovsky, A., & Anson, O. Factors related to preventive health behavior. In Cullen, J. W., Fox, B. H., & Isom, R. N. (Eds.). *Cancer: The behavioral dimension.* New York: Raven Press, 1976.

2. Best, J. A. Tailoring smoking withdrawal procedures to personality and motivational differences. *Journal of Consulting and Clinical Psychology,* 1975, *43,* 1–8.

3. Brown, E. R., & Margo, G. E. Health education: Can the reformers be reformed? *International Journal of Health Service,* 1978, *8,* 3–26.

4. Bruhn, J. G., & Cordova, K. D. A developmental approach to learning wellness behavior, part I: Infancy to early adolescence. *Health Values: Achieving High-Level Wellness,* 1976, *1,* 246–254.

5. Campbell, B. K., & Barnhund, D. D. Communication patterns and problems of pregnancy. *American Journal of Orthopsychiatry,* 1977, *47,* 134–139.

6. Dirks, J. F., Kinsman, R., Horton, D., Fross, K., & Jones, N. Panic-fear in asthma: Rehospitalization following intensive long-term treatment. *Psychosomatic Medicine, 1978, 40,* 5–13.

7. Lowery, B. J., & DuCette, J. P. Disease-related learning and disease control in diabetics as a function of locus of control. *Nursing Research,* 1976, *25,* 358–362.

8. Pless, I. B., Satterwhite, B., & Van Vechten, D. Division, duplication and neglect patterns of care for children with chronic disorders. *Child: Care, Health and Development,* 1978, *4,* 9–19.

9. Shanas, E., & Sussman, M. B. (Eds.). *Family, bureaucracy and the elderly.* Durham, N.C.: Duke University Press, 1977.

10. Shewchuk, L. A., & Wynder, E. L. Guidelines on smoking cessation clinics. *Preventive Medicine,* 1977, *6,* 130–133.

11. Simonds, S. K. Health education today: Issues and challenges. *Journal of School Health,* 1977, *47,* 584–593.

12. Wooldridge, P. J., Leonard, R. C., & Skipper, J. K., Jr. *Methods of clinical experimentation to improve patient care.* St. Louis, Mosby, 1978.

13. Zinner, E., & Hertzman, R. P.A.C.E.: A model for parent-infant support groups during the first months of life. *Clinical Pediatrics,* 1978, *17,* 396–400.

12

THE LEGAL BASIS FOR PATIENT EDUCATION PRACTICE IN NURSING*

Daniel L. Rothman and Nancy L. Rothman

Nursing's role in patient education as in all areas of health care, is defined, limited, and protected by laws. The sources of law that regulate the nurse's role in patient education are the same sources that regulate the nurse's role in all areas of health care. They are:

1. State and federal statutes enacted into law by elected officials at either the state or federal level
2. Rules and regulations promulgated by state or federal regulatory boards
3. Judge-made law based on judicial opinions in actual legal cases which set precedents for cases which are to be tried in the future.

STATUTORY LAW

One major piece of federal health legislation that deals with patient education is Public Law 93641, the National Health Planning and Resources Development Act of 1974. This act sets priorities for the formulation of national health planning goals at the federal, state, and area level. The act's purpose was to facilitate a national health planning policy. It is an attempt to counteract the inflationary trends in health care and the disparity in both the quantity and the quality of health care received by individuals in the United States, depending on their socioeconomic level and geographic location. The act attempts to coordinate planning and, very specifically, provides for consumer representation at all levels of health care planning, i.e., at all levels no less than half of the representatives of each major planning board must be consumers rather

---

*October 18, 1978

than health care providers. Ten priorities were set by Congress in Section 1502 of the act; the tenth priority speaks specifically to public education:

(10)   The development of effective methods of educating the general public concerning proper personal (including preventative) health care and methods for effective use of available health services.[11]

The fourth priority speaks specifically to nursing:

(4)   The training and increased utilization of physicians' assistants, especially nurse clinicians.[1]

Isn't it marvelous to see the area with which we are concerned, patient education, being noted by our elected officials as a priority in health care in this nation today. Isn't it encouraging to see that Congress recognizes the need for an increasing utilization of nurse clinicians. As believers in the uniqueness of the profession of nursing, the authors do not particularly like to see nurse clinicians equated with physician extenders. At least each area, state, and national plan proposed, however, is going to be evaluated as to whether it meets these needs identified by Congress as national health priorities. The funding to implement each plan will be authorized accordingly, so that behind each identified priority lies the muscle to ensure that revenue is spent to meet these identified priorities.

This piece of federal legislation identifies health education as a real need and further identifies nursing as a profession capable of appropriately intervening in the process of fulfilling this need. Our national health care delivery system is evolving from one designed to care for the ill, to one designed to keep its citizens well. It has been said that patient education is one of those things that is being fought over while nobody is doing it. Health professionals are beginning to try to identify their realm within a wellness-oriented health care delivery system. Medicine and nursing are squabbling over who has specific control or power over this new realm.

At the American Nurses Association Convention in Honolulu in June 1978, Catherine Norris, consultant in nursing in Tucson, Arizona, expressed her concern that the medical profession has received the dollar benefits from federal health care legislation and that nursing has asked for and received only limited access and control. She feels that nurses are not required to ask for access to the 80 percent of the population who are well and implies that such access is nursing's right.[2] Anita W. O'Toole of Kent State University in Ohio identified the movement of nurse practitioners into what she defines as a gap in services that has been caused by the inflationary costs of health care and the unequal distribution of physicians. Doctor O'Toole stated, "The crisis in medical care delivery has created a vacuum into which we may move!" (p 1240).[2] Nancy Risser, a medical surgical nurse with a Portland VA Hospital in Oregon, proposed that a nurse should be more involved with the goals of health care rather than the question of whether certain procedures or protocols belong uniquely to the nurse or the doctor.[2]

Is health care in the United States truly patient-oriented, or as many health care consumers have long suspected, physician-oriented? Does its major institution, the hospital, exist primarily for the education, edification, and enrichment of the medical community? While these suspicions and charges are largely unjustified, they have been engendered by certain abuses and cases of insensitivity on the part of health care providers. They have also been the impetus in the movement for formulation and enunciation of patients' rights. The formulation of patients' rights is a means of convincing the patient that the health professional looks upon him as deserving of his personal interest. The National League for Nursing, in its publication No. 11-1671 entitled "Nursings' Role in Patients' Rights"[3] includes:

Patients have the right to information about their diagnoses, prognoses, and treatment—including alternatives to care and risks involved—in terms they and their family can readily understand, so they can give their informed consent.

Patients have the legal right to informed participation in all decisions concerning their health care.

Patients have the right to appropriate instruction or education from health care personnel so that they can achieve an optimal level of wellness and an understanding of their basic health needs.

State legislatures have begun to respond to the need for a patients' bill of rights. The American Hospital Association on February 6, 1973, approved a patient bill of rights. Minnesota was the first state to require that a specific version of patients' bill of rights be posted in all hospitals and distributed to all patients. The Minnesota bill was a very watered down version of the American Hospital Association bill of rights. Other states throughout the country have passed patients' bills of rights. The authors are most familiar with the state of Pennsylvania, which published a "Patients' Bill of Rights" in the *Pennsylvania Bulletin*[4] on December 10, 1977. Of 20 rights listed, two speak specifically to patient education (p 13):

(8)   The patient has the right to full information in layman's terms, concerning his diagnoses, treatment, and prognoses, including information about alternative treatments and possible complications. When it is not medically advisable to give such information to the patient, this information shall be given on his behalf to the patient's next of kin or other appropriate person.

(20)   A patient has a right to expect that the health care facility will provide a mechanism whereby he is informed upon discharge of his continuing health care requirements following discharge and the means for meeting them.

California, Colorado, New York, and Rhode Island are other states that have specific patients' rights recognized by law.[5]

Other pieces of state legislation throughout the country that pertain specifically to nursing are commonly called nursing practice acts. In the 1970s the definition of nursing practice has been dealt with by most state legislative bodies. The changing definition of nursing has been necessary because of the changing world of the nurse. The primary purpose of the nursing practice acts is to protect the public from unqualified professionals. It is a source to which nurses need to look, however, when they are attempting to define what is nursing in their particular state. In February 1972 New York State became the first state to promulgate a nursing practice act redefining the practice of nursing by providing nurses with more professional autonomy. New York's definition reads:[6]

The practice of the profession of nursing as a registered professional nurse is defined as diagnosing and treating human responses to actual or potential health problems through such services as case finding, *health teaching,* health counselling, and provision of care supportive to or restorative of life and well-being, and executing medical regimens prescribed by a licensed or otherwise legally authorized physician or dentist. A nursing regime shall be consistent with and shall not vary any existing medical regimen.*

Pennsylvania, New Jersey, Oregon, Colorado, Indiana, Vermont, and Washington have all passed definitions that are based upon New York's definition but are individually varied.[7] The State of Washington provides:[8]

The observation, assessment, diagnosis, care or counsel, and *health teaching of the ill,* injured or infirm, or in the maintenance of health or prevention of illness of others.*

Maryland and Minnesota list functions which concern nursing. Maryland's act states:[7] " . . . the assessment, problem identification, implementation, and evaluation of . . . health needs. . . ." (p 25)

California has an entirely different approach in setting its scope of regulation for registered nurses, as it frequently does in other areas of law. Section 2725 includes the statement: " . . . the Legislature recognizes that nursing is a dynamic field, the practice of which is continually evolving to include more sophisticated patient care activities."[9] The act further states that the legislature intended to recognize that there are overlapping functions between physicians and nurses and states its intention to permit sharing the functions within an organized health care system that provides for collaboration. Patient education is not mentioned specifically but it appears to be included in Section 2725, Part A: "Direct and indirect patient care services that ensure the safety, comfort, personal hygiene, protection of patients; . . ."[9]

Every professional nurse should obtain a copy of his or her state's nursing practice act from the appropriate regulatory body and look to it for the defini-

---

*Author's italics.

tion of nursing in one's particular state and for the purpose of knowing the legal boundary concerning patient education in one's particular state.

RULES AND REGULATIONS OF REGULATORY BOARDS

Regulatory boards are generally created and empowered by federal or state legislation. Once created, a regulatory board acting with its legislative mandate may promulgate administrative regulations having the same force and effect as statutes. The regulatory body concerned with the authors' state nursing practice act is the state board of nursing known in Pennsylvania as the State Board of Nursing Examiners. Most states have regulatory boards created for the specific purpose of controlling the practice of nursing and promulgating the regulations necessary for that purpose. However, Alabama, Arkansas, California, Delaware, District of Columbia, Florida, Georgia, Hawaii, Illinois, Kansas, Kentucky, Louisiana, Michigan, Minnesota, Missouri, Montana, Nebraska, New Jersey, New Mexico, New York, North Dakota, Oklahoma, Rhode Island, South Carolina, South Dakota, Tennessee, Texas, Utah, Vermont, West Virginia, Wisconsin, and Wyoming do not give specific regulatory authority to a state board of nursing.[7] For example, within the state of New York the authority is given to the Board of Regents in the Education Law. Article 139 and the Board for Nursing in New York is advisory to the Department of Education and the Board of Regents. This is in contrast to the state of Pennsylvania, which gives the State Board of Nurse Examiners, made up of five registered nurses appointed by the Governor, the authority to issue regulations concerning the nursing practice within Pennsylvania.[10] It is becoming common to have consumer representation on professional practice boards throughout the country. Certainly, each registered nurse should obtain from his or her state board of nursing or other appropriate governmental body the rules and regulations that affect nursing practice within his or her state.

As examples of rules and regulations promulgated by the state board, the authors will share three identified areas under the responsibility of the registered nurse in Pennsylvania:[11]

(b) The registered nurse is fully responsible for all actions as a licensed nurse and is accountable to clients for the quality of care delivered.

(c) The registered nurse shall not engage in areas of highly specialized practice without adequate knowledge of and skills in the practice areas involved.

(d) The Board recognizes standards of practice and professional codes of behavior as developed by appropriate nursing associations as the criteria for assuring safe and effective practice.

These regulations are not unlike those found in other states. The statement in (d) above appears to give some legal recognition to the ANA Standards of Practice.

CASE LAW

The nurse is required to meet the same standard in the area of patient education that she or he must meet in all nursing care. Because nurses hold themselves out to be professionals with specialized training, they not only have to meet the standard of due care imposed on the laity, but are responsible for using in their professional capacity, that degree of care and skill prevalent among their peers in the locale or a similar locale in which they practice. Professional codes and standards of care proposed by the various professional groups are beginning to be accepted nationwide. When regulatory boards specifically mention standards of practice and professional codes of behavior, they are providing legal impetus for standardized nursing care requirements throughout the country.

The Code for Nurses adopted in 1950 by the American Nurses Association, which has been periodically revised and most recently copyrighted in 1976, lists as its final commitment, "The nurse collaborates with members of the health professions and other citizens in promoting community and national efforts to meet the health needs of the public" (p 19).[12] In the interpretive statement further explaining this commitment, nursing is identified as a health profession containing the largest number of health care providers. The complexity of the health care delivery systems is acknowledged as is the need for an interdisciplinary approach to health care services. The interpretive statement further speaks specifically to the relationship between nursing and medicine. The relationship is identified as interdependent; one that requires collaboration in order to meet the needs of the health care client. Nursing as a role is defined as an evolving one, requiring a collegial relationship with the physician. There remains the need to differentiate each professional's area of practice.[12] The reader may be asking, is the Code for Nurses legally binding? Codes for professionals frequently exceed the requirements of the law but are almost never less than those of the law. When a nurse fails to uphold the legal standards, the nurse may be subjecting herself to civil or criminal liability. When the nurse fails to uphold professional standards, the nurse may be subjecting himself or herself to censure by the professional organization. In addition, it can be argued that the court system has allowed the introduction of custom into evidence to aid a jury in making a determination of what standard of care is generally accepted for a health care professional or a health care institution.[13] In the case of *Darling* vs. *Charleston Community Memorial Hospital*,[14] the Supreme Court of Illinois held that evidence of the state hospital regulations, of the National Hospital Accreditation Standards, and of the by-laws of the hospital, which were introduced by the plaintiff in his personal injury action against the hospital, did not conclusively determine the required standard of care but were relevant to aid the jury in deciding what was feasible and what the hospital knew or should have known concerning its responsibility for the care of the patient. The basic dispute in this case rested upon the duty of the defendant hospital. This dispute involved:

... the effect to be given to evidence concerning the community standard of care and diligence, and also the effect to be given to hospital regulations adopted by the State Department of Public Health under the Hospital Licensing Act, to the Standards for Hospital Accreditation of the American Hospital Association, and to the by-laws of the defendant [p 256].

Justice Schaefer cited case law and quoted legal authorities:

1. By the great weight of modern American authority a custom either to take or to omit a precaution is generally admissible as bearing on what is proper conduct under the circumstances, but is not conclusive (Harper & James, The Law of Torts, Sec. 17.3, Act 977-978) [p 257].

Justice Schaefer further stated: "Custom is relevant in determining the standard of care because it illustrates what is feasible ... (Morse, Custom and Negligence, 42 Columbia Law Review 1147 (1942); 2 Wigmore More Evidence, 3rd Edition. Sec. 459, 461)" (p 257). Judge Schaefer further concluded that: "Courts must in the end say what is required; there are precautions so imperative that even their universal disregard will not excuse their omission" (p 257).

The judge's opinion clearly states in the case of *Darling* vs. *Charleston Community Memorial Hospital,* the regulations, standards, and the by-laws which were introduced into evidence by the plaintiff aided the jury in deciding what was feasible but that it did not conclusively determine the applicable standard of care, and the jury was not instructed that it did. This is why those knowledgeable in legal aspects consider standards, such as the ANA Standards of Nursing Practice, to be a two-edged sword. Certainly it is necessary for professional groups to set standards that can be used as models for the students in that profession and for the members of the profession. But it is extremely important to remember that these standards can come home to haunt the individual professional or health care institution which is unable to achieve these standards in every professional encounter. A major barrier to nurses meeting the ANA Standards of Nursing Practice appears to be the fact that so often the individual professional nurse does not control the number of people, patients, or clients assigned to her.

When one begins to evaluate what standard of patient education is required of a professional nurse, one can look as an example to the ANA Standards for Community Health Nursing Practice:[15]

STANDARD IV—PLANS FOR NURSING SERVICE INCLUDE PRIORITIES AND NURSING APPROACHES OR MEASURES TO ACHIEVE THE GOALS DERIVED FROM NURSING DIAGNOSES.

Rationale: In order to approach nursing service in a systematic manner and to achieve the goals of the nursing care plan, priorities must be established and specific nursing actions determined.

Assessment Factors:
1. Primary, secondary and tertiary measures are planned to meet specific consumer needs and are related to nursing diagnoses and goals of service.

2. Teaching-learning principles are incorporated into the plan of care. Objectives for learning are stated in behavioral terms; reinforcement is planned; readiness is considered, and the content is at the learner's level.
3. Approaches are specified for orientation of groups and communities to changing roles and life styles and patterns of health care delivery.
4. The plan includes the utilization of available and appropriate human and material resources.
5. The plan is flexible and includes an ordered sequence of nursing actions.
6. Nursing approaches are planned on the basis of current scientific knowledge.

Content is given regarding the writing of behavioral objectives and an understanding of teaching and learning principles in most Bachelor of Science in Nursing (BSN) programs throughout the country; however, it would be the unique Associate Degree (AD) or diploma graduate who would have received an understanding of the principles required in patient education. It is conceivable and logical, therefore, that if a nurse was being sued for negligence in failing to give adequate patient education, she would be compared with her peers in determining what standard of care was expetcted of her, e.g., the registered nurse who was a BSN graduate would be compared to other BSN graduates with similar experience and background, where as an AD graduate would be compared to other AD nurses.

It might be added that the contemplated legislative changes making the BSN required for entry into professional nursing practice should enhance the ability of nurses to do patient teaching.

INFORMED CONSENT

The American Hospital Association's Bill of Rights which was approved on February 6, 1972, and which was mentioned earlier, specifically states in Section 3:[16]

The patient has the right to receive from his physician information necessary to give informed consent prior to the start of any procedure and/or treatment. Except in emergencies, such information for informed consent should include but not necessarily be limited to the specific procedure and/or treatment, the medically significant risks involved, and the probable duration of the incapacitation. Where medically significant alternatives for care or treatment exist, or when the patient requests information concerning medical alternatives, the patient has the right to such information.

It is important for the nurse to understand the principle of informed consent, to what standard her state adheres, and how informed consent differs from patient education.[17]

Informed consent may be defined as a valid consent by a patient who is under no legal disability because of age or incompetency and which is based on the patient receiving an explanation of the proposed treatment from the source (treating physician) and containing all the information required by law [p 7].

The principles of informed consent are based on the right of the individual to control what happens to his body. Within the United States there are two standards for informed consent. The first, presently followed in the majority of states, holds that the patient has a right to receive the amount of information which is customarily given by the local medical community in order that the patient's consent to a procedure be considered informed consent. In the states following the majority rule, the patient-plaintiff, wishing to bring a suit on the basis that he did not give informed consent for the treatment which resulted in his injury, is required to produce an expert witness who can testify that the amount of information given to this patient fell below that standard generally accepted as custom within that local medical community.

The other standard for informed consent which is at present being followed by a minority of states within the country requires that the patient receive all the information that a reasonable man would need to have at his disposal in order to make a knowledgeable decision on whether to give his informed consent. A reasonable man is being defined here as a peer of the patient: a person of similar age, background, and experience. In our judicial system, the decision regarding what a reasonable man would require as information in order to make a knowledgeable decision is within the realm of the jury and requires no expert witness.

All the informed consent cases at this point in time have been based on informed consent for medical, as opposed to nursing treatment. The profession in whose realm or area of expertise the decision lies regarding the proposed patient treatment is the one which is obligated to obtain the informed consent. This is the area in which nurses frequently become confused, when they are called upon to have the patient sign an operative permit which generally includes a statement regarding recognition that the patient has given informed consent for a procedure. When a nurse has a patient sign this permit and witnesses it, she is witnessing the signature, an act which could be accomplished by any clerical employee who has reached the age of majority. The patient who has difficulty hearing, seeing, or reading deserves to have the statement presented to him in a manner which he can comprehend before he signs it. The nurse, being a professional employee, should be aware of hesitation by a patient and be knowledgeable enough to understand that after having signed it, a patient is able to retract his consent or change his mind. Any hesitation, change of mind, or request for additional information should be passed on immediately to the physician responsible for obtaining the informed consent. The only protection provided by having the patient sign the informed consent statement is that it may be corroborating evidence that the physician has met all the requirements within the jurisdiction which the state requires. It is important, therefore, for nurses to realize that for the purpose of informed consent for medical procedures, it is only the physician who can give the information to the patient. The informed consent, therefore, falls within a separate realm. It should not be confused with patient education with which the nurse has a great deal of responsibility in preparing the patient to gain an understanding of the patient's illness, the treatments the patient needs to perform independently, the treatments the nurse performs based on nursing decisions and nursing diagnoses, and the treatments the nurse performs based on medical diagnoses in which the nurse is responsible for carrying out the physician's orders.

A case that is still before the courts at the writing of this chapter is that of Jolene Tuma, who had her license suspended by the Board of Nursing Examiners of Idaho for having acted "unprofessionally and unethically and disrupted the physician–patient relationship."[18] Ms. Tuma, who was a clinical instructor at the College of Southern Idaho, accepted the assignment of initiating the chemotherapy for a 59-year-old terminal cancer patient at Twin Falls Clinic and Hospital in Twin Falls, Idaho. She was assisted in this by one of her AD students.[18] According to Ms. Tuma, the doctor had told the patient the night before that she, the patient, was going to die and offered chemotherapy as a last resort. When Ms. Tuma and the student arrived, the patient had been crying, according to Ms. Tuma's account. When Ms. Tuma described the side effects to the patient, the patient related to Ms. Tuma that: "She had controlled leukemia for 12 years with natural food and she felt God would perform a miracle on her behalf. She was apprehensive about the drug, but gave consent because her son wanted her to take it."[19] Ms. Tuma told the patient of alternative treatments, namely "the natural approach such as nutrition, herbs, touch therapy, and laetrile."[19] She told the patient these were not sanctioned by the medical profession.[19] The district court statement of facts that were made on behalf of Ms. Tuma stated that Ms. Tuma returned to talk with the patient and her family that evening about alternative treatment forms for cancer. While the patient was wavering in her decision and considering alternate treatment methods, the chemotherapy was interrupted for 12 hours. The patient eventually did reconfirm her consent to chemotherapy, but died several weeks later.[18] It was the physician in charge who brought charges before the Board of Nurse Examiners. This case has received a great deal of attention in the current nursing literature. In "Feedback On 'The Right to Inform'" published in the December, 1977, *Nursing Outlook,* portions of letters were published, many from leaders in the nursing field. Hildegard E. Peplau, R.N.[20] stated:

To put it more bluntly, who owns the patient? Who should control the choices and life of a patient? How should professionals view patients: as fragile china cups that break easily and must be protected, or as persons who have already survived stresses and strains and who are capable of using information to choose their own directions for living? [p 738].

Bonnie Bullough questioned: " . . . the legality of the Idaho Board of Nursing's suspension of Miss Tuma's license on the grounds that she interfered with the physician–patient relationship" on the basis that:[20]

The Idaho statute differs from most state nurse practice acts in that it does not spell out the specific grounds for suspension or revocation of the license. It does indicate that insofar as possible, those policies should conform to policies and practices of the American Nurses' Association, the National League for Nursing and the National Federation of Licensed Practical Nurse State Associations, Inc. . . . Moreover, the Idaho definition of the practice of nursing includes "observation, care and counsel of the ill" (Sec. 54-1413) [p 738].

Edith P. Lewis, R.N., Editor of the *Nursing Outlook*,[21] in an editorial addressed herself to the question, "Have we been confronted with a ruling which suggests that a major component of professionalism is to not interfere with the physician/patient relationship?" Lewis points out that the Idaho Nurse Practice Act includes as part of the definition of nursing "make judgements and decisions regarding patient's status and take appropriate nursing interventions."

The authors believe there are two problems: The first is that nurses need to have a clear understanding of informed consent and to know where their responsibility lies in this area; the second is to understand that Ms. Tuma's responsibility for patient education differed from her responsibility for informed consent to medical treatments. Therefore, she should have relayed to the physician the patient's apprehension that she picked up prior to the initiation of the chemotherapy, and allowed him an opportunity to confirm the consent that the patient previously had given.

However, the authors should warn readers that what a given nurse personally believes to be right in an ethical, moral, or "professional" sense may not be recognized as right by the courts. A nurse who suggests alternatives to the regimen prescribed by a physician in the present unsettled state of nursing law may put his or her license in jeopardy and be subject to civil and even criminal liability as well.

It is the authors' opinion that both Ms. Tuma and the physician were caught up into what we are finding to be more and more of a problem today within the health care field. There is a paranoia within each professional group to carve out an area of ownership. Boundaries between the various professional groups including medicine and nursing have become gray and hazy rather than discrete. The health team approach to patient care, with each profession having an excellent knowledge of its theoretical niche but recognizing other professions for what they have to offer the patient, can be possible only when all health professionals function in a true collegial manner, collegial being defined as: "marked by power or authority vested equally in each of a number of colleagues."[22] Communication becomes much more important when professional groups are working together with respect for each profession's expertise. The patient expects more from the health professional than from a used car salesman. He expects that for one who is interested in helping him to improve or maintain his health, the goal is better health care rather than raising profits and maintaining the supremacy of a particular professional group. Only in recent years has our health delivery system begun to be based on keeping people well rather than administering to them when they are ill.

Is patient education to become the battleground for professional jealousy? Is the ruling of the Idaho State Board of Nursing in the Tuma case symptomatic of many of the problems within nursing today? Nursing is a profession whose members have been trained in too many varied ways, and nursing has until recently not been concerned about updating our practicing professionals. We have nurses at two extremes and everywhere along the continuum: on one end, the nurse who sees herself much as the public has viewed the nurse, as hand-maiden to the physician; and on the other end, the nurse who sees herself as a completely independent practitioner, not just wanting to bring the doctor down from the pedestal and work as a team, but struggling to gain the pedestal.

The quality of health care within the United States is based on patient outcomes, and health professionals need to work together to meet the professional and legal obligations in order to teach people how to care for their health problems and maintain their health.

There have been numerous nursing research articles dealing with the effect and the effectiveness of various types of patient education. One such article, written by Linderman and Van Aernam[23] in *Nursing Research,* July-August, 1971, attempted to show that a structured preoperative teaching program reduced postoperative respiratory and circulatory complications. If this would become an accepted theory and the family of a woman patient felt she did not receive what they considered to be adequate preoperative teaching prior to her radical mastectomy and, therefore, felt the nursing staff should assume responsibility for her death following postoperative pneumonia, a suit involving the nurse's responsibility in patient education could ensue.

Once a suit is instituted, two factors become very important: adequate documentation and the degree to which the nurse defendant is covered by malpractice insurance for the claim on which the suit is based.

The records of a health care facility are generally admissible in court as evidence if the records were completed prior to the knowledge that a legal issue existed, by a person having firsthand knowledge of the facts, and written contemporaneous to the health care given. A well-documented, clearly understandable record may be an important defense in a malpractice action; for statutes of limitations being what they are, it is not unusual to find malpractice cases being tried years rather than weeks or months after the alleged incident has occurred. If patient education is an important aspect of nursing care, it needs to be documented on the patient's record. As for malpractice insurance, it is vital to any practicing nurse's financial security, professional integrity, and peace of mind.

Telling is not teaching. The patient has not been taught unless there is learning demonstrated, so health teaching needs to be recorded in terms demonstrating the outcomes of learning. Documenting the nurse has told the patient how to give insulin is not the same as documenting, "The patient correctly withdrew 12 units of NPH insulin using good aseptic techniques and injected himself at a 45° angle subcutaneously in his thigh after cleansing the area with an alcohol sponge." Patient education is certainly as important to document as medication administration, temperature, pulse, and respiration (TPR) or blood pressure.

Difficult as the concept is for readers to accept, you must understand that a nurse can be perfect and blameless and still be sued by an avaricious, frustrated, or disappointed patient. Without the protection of adequate malpractice insurance our system will impose upon the nurse-defendant the burden of hiring her own lawyer. Today $50 an hour is extremely reasonable for a lawyer's services and many hours are involved in preparing the defense of a serious case. The jury system is the best method for the administration of justice yet devised, but it is far from perfect. Under our system, the perfectly blameless nurse without malpractice insurance may be sued, incur a large bill for legal services, and lose her case and license besides. Don't let this disaster befall you. Professional liability insurance for nurses may still be obtained at reasonable rates and is in fact the biggest bargain in town.

REFERENCES

1. *Public Law 93-641,* National Health Planning and Resources Development Act of 1974, 93rd Congress, S. 2994, January 4, 1975, Title XV, Part A, Sec. 1502.
2. A.N.A. Nurses' Association Convention '78. *American Journal of Nursing,* 1978, *78,* 1231–1246.
3. *Nursing's role in patients' rights.* Publication No. 11-1671. New York, National League for Nursing, 1977.
4. Departmental issues hospital regulations. *Pennsylvania Health,* 1978, *21,* 12–13.
5. Sandroff, R. How the "patients bill of rights" makes honesty easier. *RN,* 1978, *5,* 42–47.
6. New York State Education Law, Article 139, Sec. 6902, enacted March 15, 1972.
7. Hall, V. C. *Statutory regulations of the scope of nursing practice—A critical survey.* Chicago, The National Joint Practice Commission, 1975.
8. Washington State's Business and Professions, Chapter 18.88—Registered Nurses, 18.88.030(1).
9. California's Business and Professions Code, Article 2, Sec. 2725.
10. Pennsylvania's Administrative Code of 1929, Sec. 418.
11. Rules and Regulations of the State Board of Nurse Examiners for Registered Nurses, Pennsylvania Document No. 76-2046, filed October 22, 1976.
12. American Nurses' Association. *Code for nurses with interpretive statements.* Kansas City, Mo., American Nurses' Association, 1976.
13. Annas, G. J. *The rights of hospital patients.* New York: Discus, 1975, p 29.
14. *Darling* vs. *Charlestown Community Memorial Hospital.* 211, NE, 2nd, 253–2561 (1965).
15. American Nurses' Association. *Community health nursing practice standards.* Kansas City, Mo., American Nurses' Association, 1973.
16. American Hospital Association. *A patients' bill of rights.* Chicago, American Hospital Association, 1972.
17. Rothman, & Rothman. The nurse and informed consent. *The Journal of Nursing Administration,* 1977, *12,* 7–9.

18. Idaho RN's intervention appealed in state court. *American Journal of Nursing,* 1977, *77,* 1384, 1403.
19. Letter from Jolene L. Tuma, Twin Falls, Idaho, printed under "Professional misconduct?" *Nursing Outlook,* 1977, *77,* 546.
20. Feedback on "the right to inform." *Nursing Outlook,* 1977, *77,* 738-743.
21. Editorial: The right to inform. *Nursing Outlook,* 1977, *77,* 561.
22. *Webster's seventh new collegiate dictionary.* Springfield, Mass., GTC Merriam, 1965.
23. Lindeman, C. A., & Aernam, B. The effects of structured and unstructured preoperative teaching. *Nursing Research,* 1971, *20,* 319.

APPENDIX

ADDITIONAL ASSISTS

COMMON DISTRESSES NURSES HAVE ABOUT TEACHING AND SUGGESTIONS FOR ALLEVIATION

Distress No. 1: How to start teaching and/or gain confidence in teaching.

1. Go with someone who is known to be a good teacher. Observe that person and ask questions about why each thing was done. You will disagree part of the time, but reflection will force you to come to your own reasons.
2. At first, to build confidence, teach patients who have a common learning need about which you are expert. Also of assistance is having very good teaching materials for that topic, which will limit the amount of direct teaching you need to do.
3. You will need to be persistent in continuing to work on improvement of your teaching skills. Force yourself to become expert in a second and third area of patient learning, or write your independent rationale for teaching and critique your practice against it. Some work settings are not very assistive with this kind of growth.

Distress No. 2: How to provide enough continuity of care in patient education.

1. Realize that we do not know how much continuity is really necessary to insure learning. There probably are some patients for whom continuity of teacher is more critical than for others, those who have trust in one caregiver but would have trouble establishing it with another, those for whom subject matter to be taught is not commonly understood by all staff.
2. Continuity of goals and correct responses are generally more important. Think of a variety of ways those could be obtained in your setting. Many agencies are developing standardized protocols for teaching and also providing inservice education to nurses who will be teaching. These activities can have the effect of making goals very clear and improve nurse confidence and skill in translating the patient's behavior into a judgment about whether the goals have been met.
3. One of the more serious problems in continuity is providing instruction for

as long as the patient needs it. Often the patient is in contact with health professionals primarily during one phase of illness and continues to have needs for teaching during adjustment or rehabilitation phases at home. This is primarily a structural delivery problem. You should be active in picking up needs from patients for which there may be serious consequences if they are not being met and try to change the system to provide that care.

Distress No. 3:   How to protect oneself from malpractice in the area of patient education.

1. First, be clear that the legal boundaries of a nurse's practice in patient education are not well defined, including its boundaries with the physician's practice. Because of this situation, some nurses take a conservative position regarding what they do independently and instead prefer to rely on joint interprofessional policy development, as for example, developing a diabetes education program for a hospital.
2. There are some elements of good patient education practice that can protect you, namely, evaluation of your outcomes with patients and evaluations of educational materials you use to determine whether they are effective. Since standards of patient education are not well developed at this time, it is also wise to compare the outcomes you achieve with those of other practitioners in other settings. Adequate documentation of patient education efforts and of evaluation of patient response is also essential.

Distress No. 4:   As an inservice director or head nurse, how to get all nurses to begin to do patient teaching.

1. Your goal may well be too ambitious. Some health care agencies that make a commitment to patient education do adopt the expectation that all direct care personnel will teach. Many workers already present in the system may never have learned the skills of teaching, and some of those may not want as much relationship with patients as is necessary to teach them. Unless the agency is willing to spend time for staff to practice teaching and will administratively support the expectation, not much change will likely occur. Even then, some staff will not learn, and the institution has to decide whether they are to be retained.

Distress No. 5:   How to get enough time to teach.

1. First, ask yourself honestly whether you really have some time but are not clear enough about how to teach or feel that other efforts would be better rewarded. These are skill and motivational problems in you and in the system in which you work. Some nurses do seek work situations that will support their practice of patient education. And remember that as you do patient education you become more efficient at it.

2. Realize that no system will ever meet all patients' needs for teaching, so there has to be a priority system in your institution or in your own mind to help sort out which needs will be met. Some agencies include teaching needs in their categorization of the amount and skill of care needed by various patients, so the one who is having trouble learning or for whom teaching is a very major intervention will be represented in the category system as needing more nursing care.

Distress No. 6:   How to prevent overuse of the school model.

1. Health professionals often become distressed when they realize that they have been heavily but unconsciously modeling their programs after the school model. Realize, first, that the school model works with a certain subgroup of patients, usually those who are highly schooled.
2. Use your present patient education committee or create one to make rational judgments about what outcomes should be expected from every element in your curriculum, and given those, how much instructional time is likely to be needed. If you serve heterogeneous populations of patients, this probably needs to be done for each group. Then simply test whether these outcomes (including more than just immediate goals) are being reached and whether patients are satisfied. This will give you direction on how to further alter your program.
3. Remember, discussion of the school model simply sensitizes you to the fact that not everyone can learn optimally from instruction given in that mold.

CLASSIFICATION OF PATIENT LEARNING PROBLEMS AND PATIENT RESPONSES TO INSTRUCTION

Throughout this and other books in this series, reference is made to problems in learning. Diagnostic categories related to learning have been developed as parts of overall efforts on nursing diagnosis. Since those efforts are still seen as developmental, this author's notions are presented to join in that activity.

The clinician is faced with a problem that may have very different causes and thus different interventions. An example is Kempe's[1] analysis of infant failure-to-thrive syndrome, presenting at the hospital with which he is associated:

1. Fifty percent due to maternal deprivation, often associated with severe maternal depression or rejection of the child.
2. Twenty percent are technical problems in feeding, often due to a misunderstanding or inadequate knowledge of food preparation on the part of the mother. Inadequate caloric intake can result from a rigid schedule with too much time between feedings, incorrect formula, and the wrong ratio of mixing or other technical problems such as the size of the nipple holes.

3. Thirty percent organic, comprised of 15 percent "poor feeders," often with brain dysfunction, and 15 percent other causes.

What Kempe calls technical problems constitute learning problems best addressed by teaching, although the other categories will also present learning needs. A partial classification system of patient learning problems and one of responses of patients to instruction follow.

A PARTIAL CLASSIFICATION SYSTEM OF PATIENT LEARNING PROBLEMS

Simple Cognitive
Simple terminology misunderstanding—the concept is understood
Concept has no concrete referrent—"trait" in sickle cell disease, "probability" in genetic counseling
Inaccurate notion of cause gets projected into trying to understand the treatment
Lack of simple factual knowledge, such as the value of penicillin for a cold
Inability to absorb all facts in the time allowed, with little opportunity for retrieval
Difficulty remembering information once retained

Problem Solving
Lack of identification of or consideration of an important variable, which does impact on the situation
Inaccurate probabilities of the consequences of certain alternatives
Construction of limited numbers of and inadequate quality of alternatives
Lack of an organizing idea in which to place elements, so short-term memory gets overburdened

Affective
Level of internalization and commitment requested not desired by the patient or within his behavioral repertoire
Self-expectations regarding learning ability not met

Psychomotor Skills
Cannot do some essential parts of the skill
Cannot coordinate all parts of the skill into smooth performance

Time
Teaching is not or cannot be timed to readiness
Necessity to make a decision without time to learn the full problem well enough to make an informed decision

Mastery never reached or all goals not taught because teaching conforms to time available for medical treatment

Assumption that no new learning is needed over time with long-term health behaviors.

Societal

Isolation with an unpopular view or from other people with similar problems if that company would be viewed as positive

Situations where public view is mixed, moral standards unclear, and public very unknowledgeable, so the balance of power is too strongly with the health professional

Individual does not believe in learning rational scientific thinking, and the health system is requiring it

Stigma to a disease reinforcing denial and not dealing with it

Motivation

Denial of vulnerability and/or seriousness of problem beyond the normal time for resolution

Secondary gains too strong to allow new behaviors to emerge

Lack of definite positive influences, as opposed to specific resistance

Problems Caused by Teaching Intervention (Iatrogenic)

Lack of confidence in abilities; expectations regarding patient learning may be unjustly negative

Lack of learning due to instructional environment not providing the material to be learned or direction in learning it

Inability to resolve conflicting advice and explanations given by professionals

Problems Caused by Medical Treatments (Iatrogenic)

Behaviors to be learned not reinforced when expected to be, such as treatment plan for a chronic disease that is not effective and so does not relieve symptoms when it usually should

Group/Family

Insufficient reinforcement given by the natural primary group (often the family) to cause or maintain a new behavior

Inability to identify with a new learning group and/or absence of strong natural primary group which can assist learning

Behavioral

Lack of adequate practice of the behavior

Inability to recognize cues for undesired behavior, dissociate the behavior from the cue, and reinforce new behavior

Developmental level for the skill not yet reached

Unable to take as much responsibility as is required

GLOBAL RESPONSES OF PATIENTS TO INSTRUCTION

Rejecting—Lack of trust in teacher or group teacher represents; patient may be at the wrong emotional stage of adaptation to illness

Manipulating—Such as patient falsely denying to one nurse that he has had instruction on a topic from another nurse; may be based on anger at his situation

Overwhelmed—Attention span is short; abstract and integrative thinking more limited than usual

Ambivalent—Able to understand but not committed to action; instruction sometimes brings out such ambivalence

Eager—May be eager for control over situation and to be compliant

Accepting—Wants to be cooperative and/or is resigned to doing what seems to be necessary

REFERENCES

1. Kempe, C. H. Child abuse—the pediatrician's role in child advocacy and preventive pediatrics. *American Journal of Diseases of Children,* 1978, *132,* 255-260.

Index

(*t* beside page numbers refers to tables, *f* to figures.)